STAYING HEALTHY WITH DIABETES

NUTRITION & MEAL PLANNING

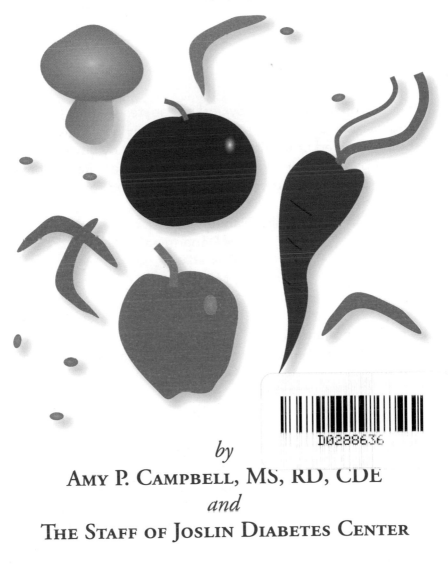

by

AMY P. CAMPBELL, MS, RD, CDE

and

THE STAFF OF JOSLIN DIABETES CENTER

Joslin Diabetes Center

ISBN: 1-879091-24-0

Published by Joslin Diabetes Center, Boston, MA

Web site: www.joslin.org

The publisher offers quantity discounts. For information, contact
Joslin Publications Department at the address above or call 617-
226-5815.

Table of Contents

Introduction
Chapter 1 What Is Meal Planning? 1
   Why Do I Need a Meal Plan? 3

Chapter 2 How Do Foods Affect Blood Glucose? 5
   Carbohydrate 6
   Protein 8
   Fat 9
   Cholesterol 11

Chapter 3 What Does a Meal Plan Look Like? 15
   Plate Method 16
   Choices (Exchanges) 18
   Consistent Carbohydrate Counting 19
   Advanced Carbohydrate Counting 21

Chapter 4 Using Food Lists and Meal Plans 23
   Food Choices At A Glance 24
   Meal Plans 24
   Until You See a Dietitian... A "Starter" Meal Plan 28
   What About Snacks? 32

Chapter 5   Meal Planning Tools .35
   Keeping Food Records 35
   Estimating Portion Sizes 37
   Label Reading 37

Chapter 6 More About Carbohydrate 43
   Can People With Diabetes Eat Sugar? 43
   Sweeteners 44
   Caloric Sweeteners 47
   Noncaloric Sweeteners 49
   Fiber And Whole Grains 51
   Tips for Increasing Fiber and Whole Grains 52
   Glycemic Index and Glycemic Load 54

Chapter 7 Heart-Healthy Eating .59

   Lipids (Blood Fats) 60

   Food Fats 62

   Food Cholesterol 63

   Plant Stanols and Sterols 63

   Soluble Fiber 64

   Tips to Reduce Your Intake of
     Saturated Fat and Cholesterol 64

   Sodium 65

   Tips for Reducing Sodium 66

Chapter 8 Tips For Cooking and Baking 69

Chapter 9 Supermarket Smarts .73

   General Shopping Tips 73

Chapter 10 Eating Out with Diabetes 75

Chapter 11 Alcohol 81

Chapter 12 Holidays and Special Occasions 87

Chapter 13 Meal Replacements .89

Chapter 14 Eating on "Sick Days" 91

Chapter 15 Vitamins, Minerals and Supplements 93

   Vitamins and Minerals 93

   Herbal and Other Dietary Supplements 95

Chapter 16 Meal Planning – Simple! 97

Joslin Food Lists 98

   Carbohydrates List 99

   Other Carbohydrates 113

   Protein List 116

   Fat List 120

   "Free" Foods List 123

   Combination Foods List 125

   Fast Foods List 127

   Food Lists for Vegetarian Meal Plans 129

INTRODUCTION

Managing your diabetes is all about making choices - and choosing what foods you will eat is one of the most important.

Each food that you eat can affect not only your diabetes, but your overall health as well. This book, together with your dietitian, will help you understand which foods you are currently eating may help keep your blood glucose levels as close to your target range as possible. You will also learn which foods you need to eat more of, or perhaps less of, if they are negatively affecting your body weight, blood cholesterol or blood glucose levels.

While there are no foods that you can't ever eat, there are foods that need to be limited to help you stay in the best of health. Research over the past decade has clearly shown that different foods affect the body in different ways. Your meal plan — your road map for good eating — will help promote a new level of wellness. By working together with your dietitian, your doctor and other members of your health-care team, you will learn to incorporate your favorite foods into your overall treatment program for good health.

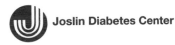 Joslin Diabetes Center

CHAPTER 1
What Is Meal Planning?

The process of choosing foods to help manage your diabetes is called meal planning. The main purpose of meal planning is to attempt to match the action of the insulin your body is producing and/or the insulin you inject with the amount and the timing of your meals and snacks.

When you go on a trip, you use a map to help guide you to your destination. You also plan special activities to make your trip a success. In a similar manner, if you have diabetes, following a meal plan will help you keep your blood glucose in your target range while at the same time allowing you to enjoy your favorite foods. In addition, if you need to lose weight or would like to maintain your current weight, a meal plan can help you meet your goal. We recommend that you see a dietitian who will work with you and provide what is called "medical nutrition therapy." This involves looking at your food and nutrition needs, and working with you to develop a meal plan that will be right for you. It is also helpful to then meet regularly with a dietitian as part of your overall diabetes care. You will no doubt have questions that need answers and your nutrition needs will change over time. There's a lot to learn about food and meal planning. If your medical goals are not being met, your dietitian may have suggestions for some changes you can make to help achieve these goals, or it may be time to change or combine medications with your meal plan. Helping you evaluate how nutrition therapy contributes to your overall diabetes treatment program is also something your dietitian can help you with.

Normally the pancreas releases just enough insulin to keep blood glucose levels within an approximate range of 60-140 mg/dl. People with type 1 diabetes must use insulin injections to replace the insulin no longer produced by the pancreas. Some

In developing a meal plan, you and your dietitian will also take into account:

▲ Your goals: Are you trying to lose weight? Gain weight? Maintain your current weight?

▲ Your medication: Are you taking insulin or oral medications? If so, how much and when does the action of your medication peak?

▲ Your medical condition: Do you have any other medical problems, such as kidney disease or high blood lipids (fats in the blood) that may influence what you should or should not eat?

▲ Your lifestyle and preferences: What kinds of foods do you like and dislike? Are you a vegetarian? When do you exercise? Do you work at night rather than during the day?

people with type 2 diabetes may have to supplement the insulin still produced by their pancreas with daily insulin injections. When your dietitian develops a meal plan with you, the question is not so much whether you have type 1 or type 2 diabetes. Rather, the question is "when and how much are you eating?" The answer will determine in part when and how much insulin you should take.

Why Do I Need a Meal Plan?

Following a carefully developed meal plan can help you consistently spread out the nutrients you need to eat for good health over each day's meals, while at the same time giving you freedom to choose what foods you want to eat. A meal plan is a guide that ensures you're getting balanced nutrition to maintain good health while, at the same time, helping you manage your blood glucose levels. By following a meal plan, you gain short- and long-term benefits that come with maintaining your blood glucose at the proper levels. You will feel better and have more energy. People who have had diabetes for many years may be susceptible to serious complications, some that can even be life-threatening. In years past, one's chances of developing such complications were high. The good news today is that following a meal plan can help reduce that risk for people with both type 1 and type 2 diabetes by helping to keep blood glucose levels in as normal a range as possible. Even if you have developed some complications from your diabetes, following a meal plan can help to slow their progression

> **A meal plan is not a diet; rather, it's a guide to help you with your food choices, and is based on the way you like to eat.**

If your goal is to lose weight...

A meal plan is especially useful if your goal is to lose weight. Being overweight affects every system in your body—and not for the better. Carrying around extra pounds makes your heart work harder and less efficiently. You'll tire quickly and become short of breath. For people who have type 2 diabetes, being overweight affects your body's ability to use insulin. Losing even a small amount of weight can not only help you feel and look better, but can also improve your diabetes control. 2. Weight loss means that you may need less insulin or oral medication to control your blood glucose. Some people with type 2 diabetes can even stop taking diabetes medication altogether when they lose weight. Other benefits of weight loss include a lower risk of getting heart disease (which is more common in people with diabetes), lower blood pressure, less back and knee pain, lower risk of some types of cancer, and lower risk of gout and gall bladder disease. That's why it's important to get on board with a healthy eating plan and regular physical activity.

The combination of a proper meal plan and a physical activity plan is the most effective way to lose weight. You may also need to change some of the behaviors that may be preventing you from shedding some unwanted pounds. Joslin Diabetes Center has developed a nutrition guideline for people with type 2 diabetes who need to lose weight, as well as for people who have pre-diabetes or who are at high risk for developing diabetes. Specifically, Joslin recommends a modest weight loss of one pound every one to two weeks. Total daily calorie intake should not be less than 1000-1200 for women, and 1200 to 1600 for men. Your doctor, nutritionist or healthcare team can help you develop a game plan based on sound medical principles for weight loss and that is realistic for you to follow.

CHAPTER 2

How Do Foods Affect Blood Glucose?

Food Groups

Before carpenters can build a house, they first must learn some basic facts about building materials. They then learn how all the pieces fit together into the framework of a building. In similar fashion, before your meal plan is developed, you must learn the basics of food and meal planning. You can then use this knowledge to develop a healthy eating style through your meal plan—a style that will help keep your blood glucose in your target range.

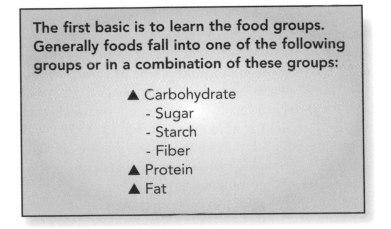

The first basic is to learn the food groups. Generally foods fall into one of the following groups or in a combination of these groups:

▲ Carbohydrate
- Sugar
- Starch
- Fiber
▲ Protein
▲ Fat

Carbohydrate, protein and fat all provide calories, or energy, which your body uses for fuel. The amount of calories you need each day depends mostly on whether you need to lose, gain or maintain your weight, and on how physically active you are. If you take in more calories than your body burns, you'll most likely gain weight. Likewise, if you take in fewer calories than your body burns, you'll lose weight. Gaining and losing weight can affect your blood glucose levels, too; blood glucose levels tend to rise when you gain weight, and drop when you lose weight.

Carbohydrate

Carbohydrate provides energy to the cells in your body. The Recommended Dietary Allowance (RDA) for carbohydrate is at least 130 grams a day for adults and children. This amount is based on the average minimum amount of glucose that is used by the brain. The two basic types of carbohydrate are **sugars** and **starches**. If you've had diabetes for a while, you may have been told in the past to avoid sugar or foods that contain sugar because it was believed that sugars would be rapidly digested and absorbed into the bloodstream, causing your blood glucose level to soar. The fact is, that if you substitute an equal amount of sucrose (sugar) for starch, your blood glucose will respond in pretty much the same way. For example, 50 grams of carbohydrate from a sugar such as maple syrup has the same effect on blood glucose as 50 grams from a starch such as bread. However, note the portion sizes: 1/4 cup maple syrup contains about 50 grams of carbohydrate whereas 3 slices of bread contain about 50 grams of carbohydrate. There are now over 20 research studies that show that when individuals choose a variety of foods containing either starches or sugars in meals, and if the total amount of carbohydrate eaten is similar, the effect on blood glucose levels will also be similar. Because foods containing either sugars or starches are broken down, or digested, into glucose at about the same rate, it is important to control *all* of the carbohydrate you eat, not just the sugars. This is the basis of *carbohydrate counting* — a meal planning method commonly used by people with diabetes to plan their food and meal choices.

Fiber is a third type of carbohydrate, although it does not affect blood glucose levels in the same way as sugars and starches. Fiber will be discussed in more detail later on.

The balance between the amount of carbohydrate foods you eat and the available insulin determines how much your blood glucose level goes up after meals or snacks. To help control your blood glucose, you need to know:

▲ what foods contain carbohydrate
▲ what average serving sizes are
▲ how many carbohydrate servings to eat

There's no magical number of carbohydrate servings that is right for everyone. Instead it is important that you work with a dietitian to determine how many servings of carbohydrate you need. Checking your blood glucose with your meter will help you see how your food intake affects your blood glucose, and if or where changes are needed. If your blood glucose levels are too high, you may need to do one of the following:

▲ eat fewer carbohydrate servings
▲ be more physically active
▲ work with your diabetes team to add or make adjustments in your diabetes medications

In addition, *Joslin* recommends that people with type 2 diabetes who are overweight or obese eat a little less carbohydrate than people who are at a healthy body weight. Studies show that eating less carbohydrate while eating slightly more protein and fat may be a better, more effective approach to losing weight than more traditional weight loss plans. In addition, eating less carbohydrate may help people with type 2 diabetes lower their risk for heart disease and improve blood glucose levels, as well. If you have type 2 diabetes and need to lose weight, approximately 40 percent of your calorie intake should come from carbohydrate. So, for example, if you were following a 1500-calorie meal plan, you would consume no more than 150 grams of carbohydrate per day. Be sure, however, not to eat less than 130 grams of carbohydrate per day.

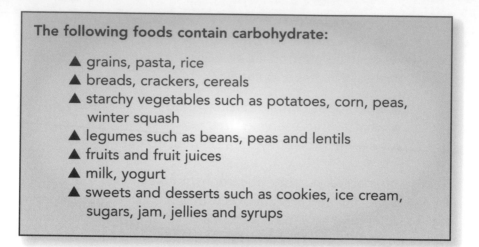

The following foods contain carbohydrate:

▲ grains, pasta, rice
▲ breads, crackers, cereals
▲ starchy vegetables such as potatoes, corn, peas, winter squash
▲ legumes such as beans, peas and lentils
▲ fruits and fruit juices
▲ milk, yogurt
▲ sweets and desserts such as cookies, ice cream, sugars, jam, jellies and syrups

Nonstarchy vegetables such as broccoli, salad greens or green beans are so low in carbohydrate and calories that they are usually considered "free."

Carbohydrate in foods is measured in grams (g). One carbohydrate serving is the amount of a food that contains 15 grams of carbohydrate. You may also hear one portion of food that contains 15 grams of carbohydrate called one "carb choice." The "Nutrition Facts" panel on food labels also lists the total grams of carbohydrate in one serving size of the food. The following are some examples of one carb choice or serving:

▲ 1 slice of bread
▲ 1 small apple
▲ 8 ounces of skim milk
▲ 1/2 cup of light ice cream

Protein

You need protein to build and repair body tissue. Your muscles, organs, bones, skin and many of the hormones in the body are made from protein. As a secondary role, protein can also provide energy for your body if carbohydrate is not available for fuel.

Meat, poultry and fish are good sources of protein. Because they are usually the primary source of protein in most people's diets, they are often referred to as "proteins." However, there are really very few foods that contain only protein. For example, most meats and meat substitutes, such as cheese and eggs, contain both protein and fat. Many of these foods have more calories from fat than from protein. Other good sources of protein such as milk, yogurt, and beans contain both carbohydrate and protein, which is why you often find them also listed on the carbohydrate list. Grains, legumes, and nuts also contain smaller amounts of protein. Tofu and other soy products, such as soy burgers, are vegetarian protein sources.

In general, most adults should limit the total amount of protein (weight after cooking) in a day to about six ounces. This is about two servings of three to four ounces and would be a serving of meat about the size of a deck of cards or the palm of your hand. For people with type 2 diabetes who need to lose weight, Joslin recommends that approximately 20 to 30 percent of calories come from protein. This means that some people could eat closer to four to six ounces of protein at a meal. However, if you have signs of kidney disease, talk to your doctor before increasing the amount of protein that you eat. For heart health and weight control, choose meats and cheeses that are low in fat. Lean beef, fish, pork, and poultry without skin are good choices. Typically, one ounce of a protein food is considered to be *one protein choice,* or *one serving.* Examples of protein servings are listed later in this chapter.

Fat

The third group of foods your body needs is fat. That's right – your body needs fat! Contrary to what you may have been led to believe, fat is not all bad. It's only when we eat too much fat or the wrong kind that it becomes a problem.

There are three types of fat found in food: *saturated fat* and *unsaturated fat* (both polyunsaturated and monounsaturated) and *trans fat*. Saturated fat is solid at room temperature. Foods that contain saturated fat include:

▲ butter
▲ shortening
▲ fatty meats
▲ whole milk
▲ cheese
▲ hydrogenated fats
▲ tropical oils, such as palm, palm kernel and coconut oils

Saturated fats raise blood cholesterol levels, which then become a part of the plaque that builds up in the blood vessels. Plaque build-up, in turn, can lead to heart disease.

Trans fat is a type of fat formed from *hydrogenation*, a chemical process that changes a liquid oil into a solid fat. The process involves adding hydrogen to the unsaturated liquid oil and changing it into a saturated solid fat. Trans fats are found in:

> Both **saturated fats** and **trans fats** can raise cholesterol levels and should be eaten in as small amounts as possible.

▲ processed foods, such as some snack foods, cookies and fast foods
▲ some stick or solid margarines

Unsaturated fats come primarily from vegetables and are liquid at room temperature. Polyunsaturated fats include:

▲ safflower oil
▲ corn oil
▲ sunflower oil
▲ soybean oil

These kinds of fat can help lower cholesterol levels. Another important type of fat is omega-3 fatty acids. This is a type of polyunsaturated fat found in fish, flax seed and walnuts. It can help lower triglyceride levels and lower the risk of heart disease.

The other kind of unsaturated fat is called monounsaturated fat. Monounsaturated fats include:

▲ olives and olive oil
▲ peanuts and peanut oil
▲ canola oil
▲ avocados
▲ nuts

Monounsaturated fat also helps to lower blood cholesterol, levels and may help to raise HDL, or "good" cholesterol levels. This kind of fat may protect against heart disease.

How much fat should you eat? Joslin's Nutrition Guideline recommends aiming for between 30 to 35 percent of your calories from fat, especially if you need to lose weight. This means that if you follow a 1500 calorie meal plan, you should aim for between 50 and 58 grams of fat each day (1 fat choice = 5 grams of fat). Be sure to choose mostly monounsaturated choices, as mentioned above.

Cholesterol

Cholesterol is often found in combination with fat in foods and acts similarly to saturated fats in the body. Cholesterol is made in the body by the liver, but is also found in some of the foods we eat. Cholesterol is found only in animal foods, such as eggs, milk, cheese, liver, meat and poultry. Eating too much cholesterol may increase your blood cholesterol levels. The goal is to limit your cholesterol intake to no more than 300 mg per day. If your LDL, or "bad" cholesterol is higher than 100 mg/dl, you may benefit from lowering your cholesterol intake to

> Only animal food contains cholesterol; fatty foods that come from plants, such as olive oil and peanut butter contain no cholesterol (but still contain fat!)

less than 200 mg per day. However, saturated fat and trans fat actually raise your blood cholesterol more than cholesterol found in food. Therefore, your first step in lowering your cholesterol level is to limit foods high in saturated fat and trans fat. And, the good news is that when you lower your intake of saturated fat (which is typically found in animal foods), you usually lower your intake of food cholesterol as well.

Remember that not all fat is "bad." We need fat in our diet to maintain healthy skin and hair, to carry fat-soluble vitamins throughout the body and to regulate our body temperature. In addition, fats are changed into fatty acids—an important source of energy. However, fat is a very concentrated source of calories. Any extra calories that your body does not use immediately for fuel are stored in the body as body fat.

"Free Foods"

You may have heard the term "free food." A free food is one that has less than 20 calories and less than 5 grams of carbohydrate in a serving. The following are examples of "free foods."
- ▲ Diet (sugar-free) sodas and beverages
- ▲ Sugar-free gelatin
- ▲ Sugar-free popsicles
- ▲ Black coffee and tea
- ▲ 1 cup raw, nonstarchy vegetables
- ▲ 1 Tbsp. fat-free cream cheese
- ▲ 1/4 cup salsa
- ▲ 2 tsp. sugar-free or low sugar jam
- ▲ 1 Tbsp. nondairy creamer
- ▲ 1 Tbsp. catsup
- ▲ Herbs, spices, seasonings

Summary

Carbohydrate, protein and fat affect your blood glucose in different ways. Most of the carbohydrate you eat, except for fiber, turns into blood glucose and the effect it will have on your blood glucose depends on the amount of available insulin (either made by your body or taken by an injection). Without enough insulin you will have high blood glucose levels. Both protein and fat also require insulin to be used by the body but have minimal effect on your blood glucose levels. Protein is used to build and repair body tissues and some protein and fat is stored for future energy needs. However, eating too much fat can cause insulin resistance, which may lead to prolonged high blood glucose levels.

How Foods Affect Blood Glucose

FOOD		FUEL
CARBOHYDRATE ~ 100% PROTEIN minimal FAT minimal	➡	Blood Glucose

NOTES

CHAPTER 3
What Does a Meal Plan Look Like?

. . . .

Ameal plan, like the sample on page 27, shows the number of servings or choices you have at each meal-time. The choices come from the food groups listed beginning on page 98. Your meal plan will likely be based on a certain number of calories as well, depending on whether you need to lose, gain or maintain your weight. The good news, however, is that you don't need to count calories as long as you aim to consume the recommended number of choices at each of your meals and snacks. Your dietitian will work with you to develop a meal plan that is realistic for you to follow. In creating a meal plan, don't think of it as a "diet." That term usually implics a drastic and temporary eating strategy often used to lose weight. Instead, the goal is to develop a healthy and life-long "eating style" that will help you control your diabetes as well as contribute to overall good health.

Using the food lists, your dietitian will help you consistently dis-tribute the nutrients you need over each day's meals, while at the same time giving you freedom to choose foods you want to eat from each list.

Your meal plan may end up looking much like the meal plan on page 27. However, there are many different methods for meal planning, and it's important to work with your dietitian to select the one that's best for you. Some common meal planning methods include:

▲ Plate method
▲ Choices (also known as exchanges)
▲ Consistent carbohydrate counting
▲ Carbohydrate counting using insulin-to-carbohydrate ratios (for people taking rapid-acting insulin before meals)

Below we'll discuss each meal planning method in a little more detail.

Plate Method

Many people find the plate method very helpful, especially when they first are diagnosed with diabetes and perhaps have not met with a dietitian yet. The "plate" can be thought of as a visual guide to help you determine how much of your plate should be filled with carbohydrate foods, protein foods and foods that contain fat.

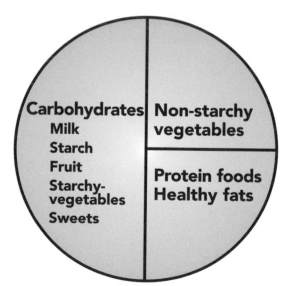

If you have type 1 diabetes, generally up to half of your plate can be filled with carbohydrate foods, a quarter of your plate with nonstarchy vegetables, and a quarter of your plate with protein and some fat.

If you have type 2 diabetes, you may need to lose some weight, and you may have a condition called *insulin resistance*. This means your body still makes insulin, but has trouble using it properly. Many people with type 2 diabetes do better losing weight and controlling their blood glucose levels by eating less carbohydrate than people without diabetes. So, on *your* plate, carbohydrate may fill up one third of your plate, nonstarchy vegetables another third, and protein and healthy fats the other third.

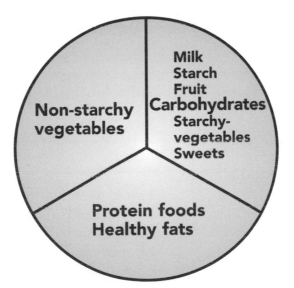

No matter what your plate looks like, it's important to aim to eat about the same amounts of carbohydrate foods each day. By doing so, you'll not only help control your portions (which can help you lose weight), you'll also help to control your blood glucose levels, too.

Choices (Exchanges)

If you've had diabetes for a while, or if you have a family member who has had diabetes for many years, you might be familiar with what used to be called the "diabetic exchanges," or the exchange system. This meal planning method was very popular up until recently, since it allowed people to vary, or exchange, the types of foods they ate within the same food group. For example, instead of eating two slices of bread (30 grams of carb), you could eat a medium potato (30 grams of carb) or two-thirds of a cup of rice (30 grams of carb). Many people still use the exchanges to help plan their meals. However, other people find this method somewhat confusing. With the help of your dietitian and a little practice, using food choices, or exchanges, can actually be quite simple and helpful in controlling your blood glucose levels.

An exchange-based meal plan for breakfast might look something like this:	
Your meal plan calls for	**You might choose**
2 starches	1 slices toast, 3/4 cup cold cereal
1 fruit	1/2 medium banana
1 milk	8 ounces skim milk
1 protein	1 boiled egg
2 fats	2 tsp. margarine

This type of meal plan is very flexible in that you can vary what you choose to eat, as long as you stay with the number of foods choices on your meal plan. For example, instead of eating toast and cereal for breakfast everyday, you might have two pancakes one day, one English muffin the next day, and one cup of oatmeal the day after that. You can then vary your fruit, milk, protein and fat choices in the same way.

If you tend to eat the same type of meals on a daily basis and would like a little more structure than some other meal planning methods, this type of meal planning approach might be helpful for you.

By the way, the choices, or exchanges, method of meal planning has led both healthcare professionals and people with diabetes to think that there is actually a "diabetic diet" that one must follow. This is really a misconception. There's no such thing as a diabetic diet, since one size certainly doesn't fit all! The best "diet" for you is a meal plan that is tailored to meet your individual needs and preferences, is something that you can stick to on a daily basis, and that helps to keep your diabetes in control while keeping you in the best health possible.

Consistent Carbohydrate Counting

Carbohydrate counting not only can help you improve your diabetes control, it offers more flexibility than the more "traditional" methods of meal planning mentioned above. Carbohydrate counting, or "carb counting" for short, has actually been around for decades. In fact, Dr. Elliot Joslin taught carb counting to all his patients many years ago.

There are really two types of carbohydrate counting: consistent and advanced. Consistent carb counting is a type of meal planning whereby you calculate, or count, the grams of carbohydrate that you eat at each meal and snack. You and your dietitian work out how many grams of carbohydrate you should eat at your meals and snacks, and that number of grams is your carbohydrate goal. Once you know the amount of carb you should be eating at your meals, the rest is easy: you can then pretty much choose what you want to eat for those grams of carb. For example, let's say your dietitian recommended you aim for 45 grams of carbohydrate for dinner. Your 45 grams of carb for dinner might look like any of these:

1 medium potato *or* 2/3 cup pasta *or* 2/3 cup rice
1/2 cup peas   1/2 cup sauce   1/2 cup frozen yogurt

Don't forget that you still have your nonstarchy vegetables, protein and fat choices to eat, as well.

So, you see that there are many options for what you can eat for 45 grams of carbohydrate. You must still be careful of your portions, including your portions of protein and fat foods, because all calories count. Yet, carb counting is appealing to many people with diabetes because it offers flexibility and variety – you need never get bored with what you eat – and lets you fit in your favorite foods, too. People often find that carb counting is much easier to do, too, compared to following an exchange-type meal plan. The key is being consistent with how much carb you eat on a daily basis. For example, if your carbohydrate goal is 45 grams of carb at dinner, but you eat 75 grams of carb instead, what will happen? Your blood glucose levels will go up! Therefore, if you keep your carb intake consistent, according to the goals your dietitian has given you, this will work along with your diabetes medication (if you take any) and physical activity to control your blood glucose levels.

> **There is no such thing as a "diabetic diet"!**

You can practice carb counting by either counting grams of carbohydrate (for example, 60 grams of carb for lunch), or by counting "carb choices." So, instead of 60 grams of carb, you'd actually be counting 4 carb choices (remember that 15 grams of carb = 1 carb choice). Either way is fine, although counting grams of carb tends to be a little more accurate, especially if you eventually start to adjust your insulin to "cover" your carb intake (see Advanced Carbohydrate Counting on page 21).

In order to carb count successfully, it's helpful to know portions of typical foods that are equal to 15 grams of carbohydrate (see the Food Lists starting on page 98). You also must learn how to read a food label for serving size and total carbohydrate, since the Nutrition Facts Label on a food package is your most accurate source of nutrition information. A carbohydrate-counting book is invaluable, as well, since many foods, such as fruit, do not come with a food label. Finally, as you start learning how to carb count, you may find that a small food scale, measuring cups and measuring spoon are helpful (at least in the beginning) to help you gauge portions. Your dietitian can show you how to properly measure and weigh foods.

Advanced Carbohydrate Counting

Y ou should understand how carbohydrate affects your blood glucose levels and the basics of carbohydrate counting. However, some people with diabetes also benefit from learning about insulin-to-carbohydrate ratios, which is the more advanced level of carbohydrate counting. This is especially important for anyone using rapid-acting insulin before meals. An insulin-to-carbohydrate ratio tells you how much rapid-acting insulin, such as lispro, aspart, or glulisine, you need to cover the carbohydrate you eat at a meal or snack. Knowing how to match your insulin dose to what you eat helps increase your flexibility in food choices and the timing of meals.

For example, your dietitian may determine that your insulin-to-carbohydrate ratio is 1:15. This means that, for every 15 grams of carbohydrate you eat at your meal, you need to take 1 unit of rapid-acting insulin to "cover" that carbohydrate. Therefore, if you plan to eat 45 grams of carbohydrate for supper, you would take 3 units of insulin for those 45 grams of carb (45 divided by 15 = 3).

If you would like to learn more about advanced carbohydrate counting, talk to your healthcare team. They can help you decide if this is the right meal planning approach for you. To learn more about advanced carbohydrate counting, refer to *The Joslin Guide to Diabetes* or talk with your dietitian.

NOTES

CHAPTER 4
Using Food Lists and Meal Plans

....

Whether you decide to use the plate method, food choices, or carbohydrate counting, becoming familiar with the Joslin Food Lists on page 98 will be very helpful for you. With some initial guidance, and the food or "exchange" lists provided in this book, you can learn to compose your meals from a wide range of choices corresponding to each of the three main food lists: carbohydrate, protein, and fat. Each list contains measured amounts of foods that are equal in nutritional value and calories. The items on a given list are interchangeable because all contain about the same amounts of carbohydrate, protein and fat, and will affect your blood glucose in a similar way.

Of course, many foods contain some combination of carbohydrate, protein and fat, and some do not fall neatly into any one food list. Pizza is a typical "combination" food, as it contains carbohydrate, protein and fat. The Food Lists included here will help you include these "combination" foods in your meal plan.

Joslin's Food Lists are similar in most ways to those provided by the American Diabetes Association. The Lists also contain a list of prepared foods, such as clam chowder, which contains a mixture of the food groups, and a list of "free" foods that can be incorporated. And beginning on page 127 is a brief list of common fast food items (the most current nutrition information on fast foods is available from each fast food restaurant or from the restaurant's website).

Food Choices at a Glance

The chart below shows the grams of carbohydrate, protein and fat in **one choice** of food from each food group. This can be helpful when trying to convert prepackaged foods into food choices for your meal plan.

FOOD GROUP	CARBOHYDRATE	PROTEIN	FAT
	Grams		
Carbohydrate			
Starch	15	3	trace
Fruit	15	0	0
Vegetable	5	2	0
Milk			
Non-fat (skim)	12	8	0
Low-fat (1%)	12	8	3
Low-fat (2%)	12	8	5
Whole milk	12	8	8
Protein			
Very lean	0	7	0-1
Lean	0	7	3
Medium-fat	0	7	5
High-fat	0	7	8
Fat	0	0	5

Meal Plans

The Joslin Food Lists are used with the meal plan developed specifically for you by your registered dietitian. You and your dietitian will consider all of the factors listed above in creating a plan. Your meal plan will look something like the *Sample Meal Plan on page 27*. At the top are your "Daily Guidelines," the total number of calories and grams of carb, protein, and fat you are allotted each day.

You will see that the form is divided into breakfast, lunch, and dinner, plus three snacks. Under each meal are listed the names of the food groups found in the food lists. On the space to the left of the food groups, your dietitian will write the number of choices of foods you may have from each food group for each meal. A "choice" is a specific portion of a food item that contains a particular number of grams of carbohydrate, protein or fat (often a combination of all three nutrients) and provides a certain number of calories. A space is also left next to each snack for your dietitian to mark in food choices you need for any snacks you eat during the day. The total number of carbs for each choice selected will add to give the total amount of carbohydrate grams that you are allowed for the meal.

In the Food Lists beginning on page 98 of this book, all the foods listed under a specific section—all vegetables for example—are equal to one "choice" (or "exchange"). One-half cup of green beans or one-half cup of carrots or one-half cup of broccoli are each one vegetable choice.

The number of choices allotted to each meal, and their distribution among the various food groups will depend, in part, on how many calories you require. An active person who needs 2500 calories per day will need more choices than someone who is trying to lose weight and needs only 1500 calories.

Once you and your dietitian have decided how to combine your nutritional and medical goals, together you will develop a meal plan of food choices. The dietitian will also write out a sample meal to show you how the meal plan works. By sticking to the number of choices on your meal plan, you will eat a consistent amount of food at each meal each day. This is very important in managing your diabetes. If you eat more than your meal plan allows, your blood glucose levels will be higher than your target level. If you take insulin or certain diabetes medications and don't eat enough, you will have too much insulin and your blood glucose levels will be lower than your target level.

Notice in the top section (right column) of the form is a space labeled "Calories." A calorie is a way of measuring the amount of energy supplied by food. Your dietitian will write in the approximate number of calories your body needs each day to balance the calories you burn. The amount is determined by your height, weight, age, gender, and level of physical activity. If you need to lose weight, the number of calories you eat will be reduced so that you burn more calories than you eat. However, you don't need to count calories; as long as you follow your meal plan you will be eating the right amount of calories.

No matter what meal planning method you decide to use, a meal plan is helpful to get you started. Eventually, with time and practice, you will become familiar with portions and the amount of carbohydrate in the foods you eat. However, you still need to pay attention to portions of non-carbohydrate foods, such as protein and fat, because they contain calories. Eating too much of any food, whether it's a carbohydrate, protein or fat, will lead to higher blood glucose levels as well as weight gain.

Be sure to let your dietitian know if you are having difficulty following your meal plan. Your meal plan is a guide for you to use to help control your diabetes. Your meal plan should be individualized, realistic and easy for you to follow. From time to time, your meal plan may need to be changed or updated, especially if you gain or lose weight, change the type of diabetes medication that you take, or change your eating schedule, for example.

Name: **JANE SMITH**

Date: **1-1-06**

MY MEAL PLAN

Daily Guidelines:
Total Calories: **1803** Carbohydrate: **221 G** Protein : **106 G** Fat: **55 G**

Meal	Sample #1	Sample #2

Breakfast Time: 7AM
4 Carb choices *or 60*
Carb grams
  2 Starch
  1 Fruit
  1 Milk
1 Meat / Protein choices
0-1 Fat choices		

Snack Time: _____		

Lunch Time: **12 NOON**
4 Carb choices *or 60*
Carb grams
  2 Starch
  1 Fruit
  1 Milk
  1-2 Vegetables
3 Meat / Protein choices
0-1 Fat choices		

Snack Time: **3 PM** **15 GRAMS OF CARB**		

Dinner Time: **6:30 PM**
4 Carb choices *or 60*
Carb grams
  2 Starch
  1 Fruit
  1 Milk
  2 Vegetables
3-4 Meat / Protein choices
1 Fat choices		

Snack Time: **9 PM** **15 GRAMS OF CARB**		

Until You See a Dietitian... A "Starter" Meal Plan

Perhaps you are wondering what you should eat while you are waiting for your appointment with a dietitian. The "plate method" will help to give you an idea of how much of each food group you should eat at each meal. (See page 16.)

Another method is to follow a temporary "starter" meal plan. The following sample meal plan can be used until you meet with a dietitian. This starter meal plan will also help you as you begin to learn more about consistent carbohydrate counting.

Breakfast

Eat 3 to 4 carbohydrate servings (choices) (remember: 1 carb choice = 15 grams of carb, so 3-4 choices = 45-60 grams of carb). Include a low-fat protein source like milk or yogurt as 1 carbohydrate serving. Typically, women should aim for 3 carb servings and men should aim for 4 carb servings at a meal.

Sample Breakfast Menus

30 grams carb (2 carb choices)

1/2 cup oatmeal 4 oz. skim milk 1 Tbsp. raisins	1/2 small bagel 1/2 grapefruit 1 Tbsp. low fat cream cheese	2/3 cup light yogurt 1/2 cup Fiber One	1 slice toast 4 oz. juice 1/4 cup low-fat cottage cheese
1/2 English muffin 1/2 banana 1 Tbsp. peanut butter	3/4 cup Cheerios 4 oz. skim milk 1/2 banana	1 low-fat waffle sugar-free syrup 1 cup berries 1 tsp. low fat margarine	2 slices "light" toast 1 cup light yogurt 1 Tbsp. low-fat marg.

Sample Breakfast Menus (continued)

45 grams carb (3 carb choices)

1 cup oatmeal
4 oz. skim milk
1 Tbsp. raisins
	1 small bagel
	1/2 grapefruit
	1 Tbsp. low fat
	   cream cheese
		1 pkt. Instant
		Breakfast drink
		8 oz. skim milk
		1 Tbsp. lower fat
		   margarine
			2 slices toast
			4 oz. juice
			1 egg

1 English muffin
1/2 banana
1 Tbsp. peanut
   butter
	1-1/2 cup Cheerios
	4 oz. skim milk
	1/2 banana
		2 low-fat waffles
		   sugar-free syrup
		1 cup berries
		1 Tbsp. lower fat
		   margarine
			2 slices "light" toast
			2/3 cup light yogurt
			1/4 cantaloupe.
			1 Tbsp. lower fat
			   margarine

60 grams carb (4 carb choices)

1 cup oatmeal
4 oz. skim milk
1/2 small bagel
1 Tbsp. raisins
1 tsp. margarine
	one 4 oz. bagel
	1 Tbsp. low-fat
	   cream cheese
	1/4 cup egg
	   substitute
		1 pkt. Instant
		Breakfast drink
		8 oz. milk
		1/2 banana
			3 slices toast
			4 oz. juice
			1 egg
			1 Tbsp. lower fat
			   margarine

3 pancakes (4 inch
   diameter)
sugar-free syrup
1 small orange
1 Tbsp. low fat
   margarine
	1 1/2 cups
	Cheerios
	8 oz. skim milk
	1/2 banana
		Blender Breakfast:
		8 oz. skim/soy milk
		1/2 cup plain yogurt
		1 Tbsp. peanut butter
		1 banana
		1/4 cup wheat germ
			2 slices whole-grain
			   toast
			2/3 cup light yogurt
			2 small tangerines
			1 Tbsp. lower fat
			   margarine

Lunch and Dinner

Eat 3 to 4 carbohydrate servings (choices) (45-60 grams).
Be sure to include some fruit and at least one non-starchy
vegetable.
Choose small portions (3 ounces) of lean meat, poultry or fish.
Include 1 or 2 servings of fat.

Sample Lunch Menus

45 grams carb (3 carb choices)

2 slices whole grain bread lettuce, tomato 1 small apple 2-3 slices lean luncheon meat 1 Tbsp. reduced-fat mayonnaise	2 slices "light" bread lettuce, tomato 10 baked chips 1/2 large pear 2-3 slices lean ham 1 Tbsp. reduced-fat mayonnaise	1 cup vegetable soup 6 saltines 17 grapes 1 oz. low-fat cheese	1 medium potato 1/2 cup broccoli 2 oz. shredded cheese 2 Tbsp. light sour cream 1/2 cup pineapple
2 cups salad 1/4 cup chick peas 1/2 cup tuna, plain 1/2 medium pita 1 cup fruit salad 2 Tbsp. light dressing	2/3 cup pasta 1/2 cup tomato sauce salad 2-3 oz. ground turkey 2 Tbsp. light dressing	1 regular fast food hamburger 1 garden salad 1 pkg. fat-free herb vinaigrette	2 cups Caesar salad 1/2 cup croutons 2-3 oz. grilled chicken 1 Tb. Caesar dressing 1/2 cup frozen yogurt

60 grams carb (4 carb choices)

2 slices whole grain bread lettuce, tomato 1 small apple 3 small gingersnaps 2-3 slices lean luncheon meat 1 Tbsp. reduced-fat mayonnaise	2 slices "light" bread lettuce, tomato 1/2 large pear 10 baked chips 2 small sandwich cookies 2-3 slices lean ham 1 Tbsp. reduced-fat mayonnaise	2 cups vegetable soup 6 saltines 17 grapes 1-2 oz. low-fat cheese	1 "wrap" sandwich with lean filling salad 2 Tbsp. light dressing 2/3 cup light yogurt
2 cups salad 1/2 cup chick peas 1/2 cup tuna, plain 1/2 medium pita 1 cup fruit salad 2 Tbsp. light dressing	1 cup pasta 1/2 cup tomato sauce garden salad 2-3 oz. ground turkey 2 Tbsp. light dressing	1 fast-food broiled chicken sandwich (no sauce) 1/2 cup frozen yogurt	1 low-fat frozen entrée garden salad 2 Tbsp. light dressing 1/2 cup sugar-free pudding

Sample Dinner Menus

45 grams carb (3 carb choices)

2/3 cup pasta 1/2 cup spaghetti sauce 2 Tbsp. Parmesan cheese garden salad 2 Tbsp. light dressing	1 cup cooked rice 1 cup broccoli 3-4 oz. baked chicken breast 1 Tbsp. low fat marg. sugar-free jello	1 cup mashed potato 1/2 cup corn 1/2 cup carrots 3-4 oz. turkey 2 Tbsp. gravy	1-4 oz. sweet potato 1 cup green beans 3-4 oz. broiled fish 1/2 cup applesauce 1 Tbsp. lower fat margarine
1 cup veg. soup 2 slices bread 3 oz. tuna lettuce, tomato 1 Tbsp. reduced-fat mayonnaise	2 tortillas 1/2 cup refried beans 1/2 cup salsa lettuce, tomato 2 Tbsp. light sour cream	2/3 cup brown rice 1 cup stir-fry vegetables 3-4 oz. light tofu 1/2 cup light ice cream	1 hamburger bun 3-4 oz. lean hamburger patty lettuce, tomato 10 baked french fries

60 grams carb (4 carb choices)

1 cup pasta 1/2 cup spaghetti sauce 2 Tb. Parmesan cheese garden salad 2 Tbsp. light dressing	1 cup cooked rice 1 cup broccoli 3-4 oz. baked chicken 1 small apple 1 Tbsp. lower fat margarine	1 cup mashed potato 1/2 cup corn 1/2 cup carrots 1 small roll 3-4 oz. turkey 2 Tbsp. gravy	1-4 oz. sweet potato 1 cup green beans 3-4 oz. broiled fish 1/2 cup applesauce 8 oz. skim milk 1 Tbsp. low fat margarine
2 cups vegetable soup 2 slices bread 3-4 oz. tuna lettuce, tomato 1 Tbsp. reduced-fat mayonnaise	2 small tortillas 1/2 cup refried beans 1/3 cup rice 1/2 cup salsa lettuce, tomato 2 Tbsp. light sour cream	1 cup brown rice 1 cup stir-fry vegetables 3-4 oz. light tofu 1/2 cup light ice cream	1 hamburger bun 3-4 oz. lean hamburger patty lettuce, tomato 10 baked french fries 1/2 cup pineapple

Sample Dinner Menus (continued)

75 grams carb (5 carb choices)

1 cup pasta 1 cup spaghetti sauce 2 Tbsp. Parmesan cheese salad 2 Tbsp. light dressing	1-1/3 cups cooked rice 1 cup broccoli 3-4 oz. baked chicken 1 small apple 1 Tbsp. lower fat margarine	1 cup mashed potato 1 cup corn 1 cup carrots 1 small roll 3-4 oz. turkey 2 Tbsp. gravy	1-4 oz. sweet potato 1 cup green beans 3-4 oz. broiled fish 1/2 cup applesauce 3 small gingersnaps 8 oz. skim milk 1 Tbsp. lower fat margarine
2 cups vegetable soup 2 slices bread 3-4 oz. tuna lettuce, tomato 1/2 cup sugar-free pudding 1 Tbsp. reduced-fat mayonnaise	2 small tortillas 1/2 cup refried beans 2/3 cup rice 1/2 cup salsa lettuce, tomato 2 Tbsp. light sour cream	1-1/3 cups brown rice 1 cup stir-fry vegetables 3-4 oz. light tofu 1/2 cup light ice cream	1 hamburger bun 3-4 oz. lean hamburger patty lettuce, tomato 10 baked french fries 1/2 cup pineapple

What About Snacks?

Years ago, people with diabetes were usually told to eat two to three snacks each day to prevent blood glucose levels from going too low between meals. Today, however, thanks to newer insulins and diabetes medications, many people with diabetes can avoid having to eat a snack. Some people find snacks inconvenient, especially while working, and people who are trying to lose weight often dislike having to consume extra calories when they're not hungry.

Of course, like many people with diabetes, you might prefer to have at least one snack during the day, particularly if, for example, you eat lunch at noontime and dinner is not until 6:00 pm. You might simply get hungry!

Talk with your dietitian as to whether you should include snacks in your meal plan. If your goal is to lose weight, you might decide that having some raw vegetables or sugar-free gelatin is enough to satisfy those hunger pangs mid-afternoon. Your dietitian will take into account your blood glucose levels, type of diabetes medications, meal schedule and activity level (along with your own preferences!) when deciding to fit snacks into your meal plan.

Snacks
If you need a snack, eat 1 to 2 carbohydrate servings (choices) (15-30 grams carb). Women should aim for 1 carb serving and men should aim for 1-2 carb servings for snacks.

And don't forget to choose healthful snacks, such as fruit, low-fat yogurt or whole grain crackers, rather than potato chips, cookies or other high-fat snack foods.

Use the list below for snack ideas.

Snack Choices

One Carbohydrate

The foods in this section each contain about 15 grams of carbohydrate and 60-80 calories per serving. Items marked with an asterisk also have one (*) or two (**) servings of fat.

Bread (1 1-oz. slice)
Pita (1/2 of a 6" pita)
English muffin (1/2)
Bagel (1/4 of a 4-oz. bagel)
Bread sticks (2)
Unsweetened cereal (3/4 cup)
Granola, low-fat (1/4 cup)
Rice cakes/Popcorn cakes (2 large)
Pretzels (2 rods or 3/4 ounce)
Tortilla chips (6-12 or 1 ounce)**
Popcorn (3 cups air popped or low fat
    microwave)
Melba toast (4 slices)
Goldfish (43)
Snack chips, baked (tortilla, potato) 15-20
Ak-Mak (10 crackers, 2 oz)
Saltine-type crackers (6)
Crackers, round butter type (6)*
Oyster crackers (24)
Mini Stoned Wheat Thins (14)
Ginger snaps (3)
Graham crackers (3 squares)
Granola bar (1)*
Animal crackers (8)
Vanilla wafers (5)*
Fig Newtons (2)
Rice Krispie Treat (1)
Angel food cake (1/12th of a cake)
Fresh fruit - small apple, orange,
    banana
Grapes (17)
Raisins (2 Tbsp.)
Fruit juice bar, frozen,100% juice
    (1- 3 oz bar)
Yogurt, frozen, low-fat (1/2 cup)
Ice cream, light (1/2 cup)*
No-sugar-added fudgesicle (2)
Light-style yogurt (2/3 cup)
No Sugar Added hot chocolate (8 oz)
Sugar-free pudding (1/2 cup)

One Protein

The foods in this section each contain about 5-8 grams of protein and 35-100 calories per serving. Lean choices have 3 grams or less of fat per serving.

Cheese, low-fat (1 ounce)
Parmesan cheese, grated (2 Tbsp.)
Cottage cheese, low-fat (1/4 cup)
Ricotta cheese, low-fat (1/4 cup)
Laughing Cow Light cheese (1 wedge)
Tuna, canned in water (1/4 cup)
Shrimp, 1 ounce (about 4 medium)
Egg, hard boiled (1)
Peanut butter (1 Tbsp.)**
Lean meat or poultry (1 ounce)
Hot dogs, low-fat (1)
Luncheon meat, low-fat (1 ounce)

One Fat

The foods in this section contain about 5 grams fat and 45 calories per serving.

Avocado, medium (1/8th)
Olives, black (8 large)
Olives, green (10 large)
Peanuts (10)
Almonds (6)
Pumpkin, sunflower seeds (1 Tbsp.)
Tahini, or sesame paste (2 tsp.)

CHAPTER 5
Meal Planning Tools

....

Keeping Food Records

P aying attention to what you eat is important, especially when you have diabetes. Many people find that keeping food records helps them do this. If you haven't met with a dietitian, it's a great idea to write down what and when you eat and drink for three days. Take the record to your appointment with the dietitian. That way you and your dietitian can develop your meal plan around your usual eating habits and lifestyle as much as possible.

Once you start following your new meal plan, your dietitian will likely ask you to continue keeping a food record or to keep track of the "servings of carbohydrate" you eat (1 serving = 1 choice or 15 grams of carb). To do this, write down the time, and everything you eat and drink, each day. Try to estimate the amount or serving size of each food and drink. If you are just keeping track of carbohydrate servings, use the Food Choice Lists at the end of this book. You might find it helpful to keep the results of your blood glucose checks along with your food or carbohydrate record. On the next page is an example of a food record.

Do you have to keep a food record every day, for the rest of your life? Not necessarily. Again, it's helpful to keep a food record when you first begin to follow a meal plan or start counting carbs. Once you're in a routine and you're comfortable with how much carb you should be eating, you probably won't have to keep a record as often. However, if you have unexplained high or low blood glucose levels, if you start to gain weight, or if you experiment with eating different types of foods, for example, you will find that keeping a food record, even for just a few days in a row, is an invaluable tool to assess how well you are in control of your diabetes.

Sample Food Record

	BREAKFAST		SNACK	LUNCH		SNACK	DINNER		SNACK
	Before	After		Before	After		Before	After	
Time									
BG									
Food and Amount DAY 1	Carb_____gm			Carb_____gm			Carb_____gm		
Time									
BG									
Food and Amount DAY 2	Carb_____gm			Carb_____gm			Carb_____gm		
Time									
BG									
Food and Amount DAY 3	Carb_____gm			Carb_____gm			Carb_____gm		

BG - Blood Glucose

Estimating Portion Sizes

Portion control is a key factor in meal planning. If you plan to eat one cup of cooked pasta (which would be 3 carb choices or 45 grams of carb), how do you know you're eating one cup and not two or three cups? The only way to really be sure is to weigh and measure your foods. By doing so, you'll be able to train your eye to gauge portions, and in turn, will have better blood glucose control. In your own kitchen it's quite easy and convenient to measure and, if necessary, weigh foods. A measuring cup or scale is the best way to keep close tabs on your portion sizes. Always weigh or measure foods *after* cooking.

Use a food scale that measures in ounces for weighing foods such as:

▲ meat, poultry, fish and cheese

Use a measuring cup for portioning out dry foods such as:

▲ cereal, pasta, and rice.

Use a liquid measuring cup for liquids, such as:

▲ milk and juice

Use measuring spoons (not your regular spoons) for foods eating in smaller amounts, such as:

▲ peanut butter, mayonnaise and salad dressing.

With practice, you will be able to estimate accurately and you will not need to use the scale or measuring cups all the time.

If you're like many people, a lot of your meals are probably eaten outside of your home. In this case, your hand can be a "handy" tool to help you determine portion sizes. Men may need to estimate down a little bit, since the measures below are based on a woman's hand of average size. The following tips for using your hand will make it easier to estimate portions:

▲ Your *fist* is about the size of one cup.

▲ Your *palm* is about the size of 3 ounces of cooked meat; this is also the size of a deck of cards.

▲ Your *thumb* is about one ounce of cheese, or one table spoon of salad dressing or peanut butter.

▲ Your *thumb tip* (the top joint of your thumb) is about one teaspoon. One teaspoon equals one serving of fat, such as butter, margarine, mayonnaise, or oil.

▲ Your *whole hand* is a handful of about one to two ounces of a snack food (not a heaping handful). About three handfuls of popcorn equals one ounce (1 carbohydrate serving). For pretzels, two handfuls equals 3/4 ounce (1 carbohydrate serving).

Some people find it easier to visualize portion sizes. Try to picture the following:

▲ 1 ounce of meat looks like a matchbox

▲ 1 ounce of cheese is about the size of a ping-pong ball

▲ 1 tablespoon of peanut butter is about the size of a walnut

▲ 1 cup of fruit is about the size of a baseball

▲ A medium apple or orange is about the size of a tennis ball

▲ A bunch of grapes equal to a 1/2 cup serving is about the size of a light bulb

▲ A medium potato is about the size of a computer mouse

If you eat away from home a lot, your idea of a serving tends to increase without you noticing. So when you're at home, it is always a good idea to periodically check your portions and keep your portion estimation skills strong.

Label Reading

Food labels are another important tool to help you know what you are eating. If you look at the packaging of almost all foods in your grocery store, you'll find detailed information about nutrition on the "Nutrition Facts" panel. However, often the problem is too much information and you may not be sure what information on the label will be most useful for managing your diabetes. The Nutrition Facts food label on this page is a typical food label. The steps on the following pages will help you decide how to "count" the food described on this label.

Whole Grain Cereal

Nutrition Facts

Serving Size: 1 cup (53g/1.9 oz)
Servings per Container: About 8

Amount Per Serving

Calories 190 Calories from Fat 25

	% Daily Value*
Total Fat 3g	**5%**
Saturated Fat 0g	**0%**
Trans Fat 0g	
Cholesterol 0mg	**0%**
Sodium 95mg	**4%**
Potassium 300mg	**9%**
Total Carbohydrate 36g	**12%**
Dietary Fiber 8g	**32%**
Soluble Fiber 3g	
Insoluble Fiber 5g	
Sugars 3g	
Protein 4g	**14%**

Vitamin A 0%	Vitamin C 0%
Calcium 4%	Iron 10%
Phosphorus 10%	Magnesium 10%
Copper 8%	

*Amount in Cereal. One half cup of fat free milk contributes an additional 40 calories, 65 mg sodium, 6g total carbohydrates (6g sugars), and 4g protein.

**Percent Daily Values are based on a 2,000 calorie diet. Your daily values may be higher or lower depending on your calorie needs.

	Calories:	2,000	2,500
Total Fat	Less Than	65g	80g
Sat Fat	Less Than	20g	25g
Cholesterol	Less Than	300mg	300mg
Sodium	Less Than	2,400mg	2,400mg
Potassium		3,500mg	3,500mg
Total Carbohydrate		300g	375g
Dietary Fiber		25g	30g
Protein		50g	65g

Calories per gram:
Fat 9   •   Carbohydrate 4   •   Protein 4

INGREDIENTS: Soy Grits, Hard Red Winter Wheat, Long Grain Brown Rice, Whole Grain Oats, Barley, Rye, Buckwheat, Sesame Seeds, Evaporated Cane Juice Syrup, Corn Meal, Corn Flour, Soy Protein, Wheat Bran, Oat Flour, Corn Bran, Honey, Natural Flavors, Calcium Carbonate, Salt

CONTAINS SOYBEAN AND WHEAT INGREDIENTS

Serving Size

Begin by looking at the *Serving Size*. Is this the amount you plan to eat? This is important because the nutrition information on the label is linked directly to the serving size. If you typically eat more than what is called "one serving," you will need to account for the extra amount.

Total Carbohydrate

Next, focus on the *Total Carbohydrate*. This number is used to determine the number of carbohydrate servings in the serving size. The important number to remember is:

15 grams carbohydrate always equals 1 carbohydrate serving (choice)

Therefore, using the information on the Nutrition Facts Food Label on page 39, a serving is 1 cup and contains 36 grams of carbohydrate. To determine how to "count" 1 serving of the cereal described in the food label, divide the 36 grams of carbohydrate by 15 (15 grams carbohydrate in one carbohydrate serving), which is equal to about 2-1/2. This means that one cup of cereal is counted as 2-1/2 carb choices. Ignore the *sugars* amount as it is already counted within the total carbohydrate; don't add the grams of sugars to the grams of total carbohydrate. Note that the sugars and dietary fiber are indented and in lighter print than the total carbohydrate. Often people assume the sugars are simply the added sugars. But in fact the sugars include both added and naturally occurring sugars, such as lactose in milk and fructose in fruit, found in the food.

When counting carbohydrate, most people can also ignore the *dietary fiber* amount as well. However, for individuals trying to be very precise with the carbohydrate amount, for example, when determining an insulin-to-carbohydrate ratio for more "advanced" carbohydrate counting, if the dietary fiber amount is greater than 5 grams, you can subtract it from the total carbohydrate grams. Dietary fiber is not absorbed, but it is unlikely that 5 to 10 grams of fiber will have much effect on your blood glucose level unless you eat more than one serving. Fiber does have many health benefits, however, which means you should aim to include high-fiber foods at each of your meals.

Some labels may also list *sugar alcohols*, which are used in some foods as sweeteners. In general, about half of the grams of sugar alcohols are digested. Just as for fiber, when counting carbohydrate you can generally ignore the sugar alcohol amount. However, when determining an insulin-to-carbohydrate ratio, if the sugar alcohol is more than 10 grams, you can subtract half of the amount from the total carbohydrate grams.

Net-carb, *low-carb*, and *impact carb* are relatively new phrases on labels. They are currently not defined by the Food and Drug Administration (FDA), although it is working on defining them now. These terms were created by companies to give their products more "shelf appeal." Currently the best advice is that consumers should not be fooled by promises on wrappers. Calories still count and these special "low-carb" food products are not calorie-free and can still affect your blood glucose levels.

Total Fat

The Total Fat on the label is the total grams of fat in a serving of this food — *saturated*, *monounsaturated*, *polyunsaturated* and *trans fats*. It's best to choose foods made from *monounsaturated* or *polyunsaturated* fats. Avoid products that contain large amounts of *saturated* fats and keep *trans* fats to as small an amount as possible.

Total fat grams per day should be about 40 to 70 grams for women and 60 to 90 grams for men. A food can be labeled low-fat if it has 3 grams or less of fat in one serving. A low saturated fat food has no more than 1 gram of saturated fat per serving. Look at the total grams of fat in one serving size and select foods with:

▲ 3 or less grams of fat for every 15 grams of carbohydrate
▲ 3 grams of fat for every 7 to 8 grams of protein (or one ounce of a protein food)
▲ 1/3 or less of the total fat as saturated fat

Sodium

Sodium is listed in mg (milligrams) per serving. Choose foods that have less than 400 milligrams in a single serving or less than 800 milligrams for convenience food or meal entrées.

Learn the Label Lingo

Label terms that you see on a food box or package have standard definitions set by the Food and Drug Administration (FDA). Here are some of the most common terms you will see:

▲ Fat-free   Less than 0.5 gram of fat per serving

▲ Low-Fat   3 grams fat or less per serving

▲ Low Saturated Fat   1 gram of saturated fat or less per serving

▲ Low Cholesterol   20 mg or less and 2 grams or less of saturated fat per serving

▲ Low-Sodium   140 milligrams sodium or less per serving

▲ Low-Calorie   40 calories or less per serving

▲ Lean   Less than 10 grams of fat, 4 grams of saturated fat, and 95 mg of cholesterol per serving

▲ Light   1/3 fewer calories or 1/2 less fat than the regular version; or no more than 1/2 the sodium of the higher-sodium version

▲ Reduced   25% less of a specific nutrient, or 25% fewer calories than the regular version

▲ Sugar-free   Less than 0.5 gram of sugar per serving

▲ No Sugar Added   No sugar added during processing

CHAPTER 6
More About Carbohydrate

....

Can People With Diabetes Eat Sugar?

Nutrition guidelines issued in 1994 by the American Diabetes Association say it's okay for people with diabetes to substitute sugar-containing foods for other carbohydrates as part of a balanced meal plan. The guidelines note that there is relatively little scientific evidence to support the belief that simple sugars are more rapidly digested and absorbed than starches and therefore more apt to produce high blood glucose levels. The guidelines recognize that, when total calories and nutrients are considered, sugar can be eaten in modest amounts. What is important is the *total amount* of carbohydrate in the diet, rather than its source. This is where a carbohydrate counting meal plan comes in. Once you know how to count carbohydrates, you'll be able to fit any food, including sugar, into your meal plan.

High-sugar foods are more concentrated in carb; therefore, for a given amount of carb, the portion size is smaller for a high-sugar food than for a low-sugar food. Are you able to control your portion size, or are you likely to overeat? High-sugar foods might not be a good choice if they will tempt you to eat more.

If you would rather eat larger portions, select low-sugar choices. Look at the differences in portion size for equal amounts of carb in these cereals!

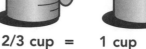

| 1/3 cup = | 1/2 cup = | 2/3 cup = | 1 cup |
| Raisin Bran | Cornflakes | Cheerios | Puffed Wheat |

If you do want a "sweet," make a low-fat choice, such as low-fat frozen yogurt, gingersnaps, fig bars or graham crackers and substitute it for foods containing an equal amount of carb in your meal plan.

Sweeteners

Sweeteners can be divided into those that contribute calories (called *nutritive* or *caloric sweeteners*) and those that contribute few, if any, calories, called either noncaloric or nonnutritive sweeteners. If you have diabetes, there is a wide range of sweeteners that will fit into your eating plan. Not all sweeteners are alike—they can have a different effect on your blood glucose. The table, *Sugars, Sweeteners, and Sweets*, on the following page lists most of the sweeteners available today and the common or brand names by which they are known.

Sugars, Sweeteners, and Sweets

Caloric Sugars, Sweeteners, and Sweets	Common Names	Comments/Applications
Carob	Carob flour Carob powder Carob chips	75% sucrose, glucose, and/or fructose. Tastes like chocolate.
Chocolate	Bittersweet Bitter Milk chocolate	40% to 43% sucrose
Fructose	Fruit sugar Levulose	100% fruit sugar
Glucose	Corn sugar Dextrose Grape sugar	Not as sweet as sucrose
Honey	Creamed honey Honeycomb	About 35% glucose, 40% fructose plus water
Lactose	Milk sugar	50% glucose, 50% lactose. Not as sweet as sucrose
Maltose	White crystalline sugar formed from starches	100% glucose. Not as sweet as sucrose
Molasses	Black strap Golden syrup Refiner's sugar	50% to 75% sucrose and invert sugar

Sucrose	Beet sugar Brown sugar Cane sugar Confectioner's sugar Dehydrated cane juice (Sucanat) Invert sugar Powdered sugar Raw sugar Table sugar Turbinado	50% glucose, 50% fructose
Sugar alcohols (polyols)	Ducitol Isomalt Maltitol Mannitol Sorbitol Xylitol Hydrogenated starch hydrolysate	Add sweetness and bulk to foods. Not as sweet a sucrose; have about half the calories as other sugars because they are not completely absorbed. May cause abdominal pain, cramping, gas, bloating and diarrhea, especially in children.
Syrups	Corn syrup Corn syrup solids and/or fructose High fructose syrups Honey maple syrup Molasses Sugar cane syrup Sorghum syrup	Primarily glucose
Acesulfame-K	Sweet One Sunette	200 times sweeter than sucrose. Can be used in baking and cooking.

Aspartame	Equal NutraSweet Sweet Mate	180 times sweeter than sucrose. Loses sweetening effect when heated. Prolonged cooking at high heat may result in loss of some sweetness.
Neotame		8,000 times sweeter than sucrose. Only very small amounts are needed to sweeten foods and beverages. Can be used alone or in combination with other noncaloric or caloric sweeteners.
Saccharin	Sweet 'n Low Sugar Twin Sweet Magic Sucaryl	375 times sweeter than sucrose. Can be used in baking and cooking.
Sucralose	Splenda	600 times sweeter than sucrose. Can be used in cooking or baking. It pours, measures, and bakes like sugar.

Caloric Sweeteners

Caloric sweeteners are carbohydrates and they do affect your blood glucose levels. Most of them contain 4 calories per gram, just like other carbohydrates. This means you need to count caloric sweeteners just the same as you count other carbohydrate foods. Caloric, or nutritive, sweeteners contribute calories without any other nutritional value, so just like everyone else, people with diabetes should be careful of how much they eat or drink of sweetened foods.

One simple way to keep "sweetness" in your meals without adding extra amounts of carbohydrate is to cut back on the amount of sugar you use. With most recipes you can reduce the sugar by at least one third without changing the taste and texture. For example, if a recipe calls for 1 cup of sugar, use 2/3 cup instead, and next time try 1/2 cup.

Be aware! "Sugarless," "sugar-free" and "no sugar added" usually mean that sucrose (table sugar), dextrose, corn syrup, honey and other sugars have been replaced with sweeteners known as sugar *alcohols* or *polyols* that cause a slightly lower rise in blood glucose. This does not mean that these foods are necessarily better for people with diabetes, as they are usually not reduced very much in calories. And, many people don't realize that "sugar-free" foods still contain carbohydrate – often, just as much carbohydrate as the "regular" version! These foods may even contain higher amounts of fat, which can increase their calories per serving. Bloating, gas, diarrhea and stomach upset are also common side effects of the sugar alcohols.

There are some general guidelines to help you do carbohydrate counting with sugar alcohols.

▲ Sugar alcohols are usually combined with other carbohydrates, therefore subtract *half* of the sugar alcohol's grams from the total carbohydrate grams and count the remaining carbohydrate grams.

▲ If ALL the carbohydrate and calories are from sugar alcohols, and the carbohydrate grams are less than 10 grams per serving, it is considered a free food.

▲ If ALL the carbohydrate is from sugar alcohols, and the carbohydrate grams are over 10 grams per serving, divide in half and count half as grams of carbohydrate.

Noncaloric Sweeteners

There are now five noncaloric sweeteners approved for use. Four are listed in the table on the following page. Neotame is the latest noncaloric sweetener to be approved by the Food and Drug Administration (FDA). Other than saccharin, which was on the market before the FDA established the food additive approval process, the others were all approved through FDA's rigorous safety process. Saccharin, which in very large quantities was linked to cancer, was dropped from the FDA's cancer-causing chemical list in 2000, and the label of saccharin-containing products no longer requires a health warning. Articles are often circulated on the Internet questioning the safety of aspartame. Aspartame has been the subject of over 200 studies since 1965. These studies have concluded that eating products sweetened with aspartame is not associated with any adverse health effects.

After extensive testing, all approved noncaloric sweeteners were determined to be safe for the general public, including people with diabetes, and during pregnancy and lactation. The following recommendations are set by the FDA for Acceptable Daily Intake (ADI) and include a 100-fold safety factor. The World Health Organization's Joint Expert Committee on Food Additives has set the ADI for saccharin.

Noncaloric Sweeteners

	ADI* (mg/kg body weight)	Average amount (mg) in 12-oz can of soda**	Cans of soda to reach ADI for 100 pound person	Amount (mg) in a packet of sweetener	Packets to reach ADI for a 100 pound person
Acesulfame-K	15	40+	17	50	13
Aspartame	50	200	11	35	63
Saccharin	5	140	1.6	40	6
Sucralose	5	70	3.2	5	45

*Acceptable Daily Intake
**This number represents an average; different brand names and fountain drinks may have varied amounts of sweeteners.
+ Based on the most common blend with 90-mg aspartame.
Table adapted from: *American Diabetes Association Guide to Medical Nutrition Therapy for Diabetes*, 2005.

The benefit of noncaloric sweeteners is that they can be used in foods and beverages without adding carbohydrate or calories. A major advantage is the use of these sweeteners in sodas and soft drinks. Consider that a 12-ounce regularly sweetened soda contains about 155 calories and 40 grams of carbohydrate (the equivalent of 10 teaspoons of sugar). A soda sweetened with a noncaloric sweetener, such as aspartame, contains 0 calories and 0 grams of carbohydrate. According to the table above, a soda sweetened with Aspartame would contain 200 mg of it and a 100 lb person could drink 11 cans before exceeding their Daily Intake (ADI). Often the first step in improving glucose levels is to substitute diet drinks for regular sodas and soft drinks.

You can't totally substitute noncaloric sweeteners for sugar in baking. Why? Because sugar provides bulk as well as sweetness to these recipes. In some recipes, you can replace some of the sugar with a noncaloric sweetener. Adding nutmeg, cinnamon, vanilla, or almond extract in place of some of the sugar will also add "sweetness" to your recipes. These flavorings give foods a sweet taste without adding sugar or calories.

Fiber and Whole Grains

Earlier, you learned that fiber is a type of carbohydrate, just like starches and sugars. Fiber is the structural portion of fruits, vegetables, grains, nuts, and legumes that cannot be digested or absorbed by your body. Therefore, fiber does not provide calories. Some fibers add "bulk" to your meals, helping you feel full. Other fibers have a laxative effect on the digestive system. Common sources of fiber are wheat, corn, or oat bran; legumes (cooked dried peas and beans); nuts; and vegetables and fruits, especially when raw.

Very large amounts of fiber, approximately 50 grams per day, have been shown to improve glucose, lipid (fat), and insulin levels. Because the average fiber intake in the United States is about 10 to 13 grams per day, some people with diabetes may find it challenging to consume enough fiber on a regular basis to improve their blood glucose control. However, there are other benefits of eating a diet high in fiber and whole grains, including a lower risk for heart disease and some types of cancer; improved digestive health; and even weight control. In addition, foods high in fiber typically contain more of the important vitamins and minerals that may be missing in refined or processed foods.

Fiber and whole grains go hand-in-hand. Whole grains include all three parts of the grain—the bran, germ, and endosperm. The fiber, vitamins, minerals and hundreds of phytonutrients (health-protective substances in plant foods) found in grains work together to help protect against heart disease and diabetes, and may help with blood glucose control. The best way to identify whole grain foods is to look at the ingredient list on the package. Look for foods with the whole grain ingredient listed first—for example, whole-wheat flour, whole oats, whole grain corn, or brown rice.

Tips for Increasing Fiber and Whole Grains

The goal is to increase your fiber intake to between 20 and 35 grams per day. Joslin recommends aiming for closer to 50 grams of fiber per day, if possible, especially if you have type 2 diabetes and need to lose weight. While this can be challenging to do, eating high-fiber cereals, such as All Bran, and using fiber supplements can help you reach this goal. If you're not used to eating much fiber, you should increase your intake gradually (by 3-5 grams per day) to allow your digestive system time to "adjust." Eating too much fiber at once can lead to gas, cramps and even diarrhea. Also, be sure to increase your fluid intake as you increase your fiber intake in order to avoid constipation.

Here are ways you can increase the fiber content of your meals:

▲ Dietary fiber is listed right under Total Carbohydrate on the Nutrition Facts Label. Foods that are an excellent source of fiber have 5 grams or more per serving and good sources of fiber are foods with 2-1/2 to 5 grams per serving.

▲ Choose foods with a high-fiber content, such as whole-grain cereals, breads and crackers; grains such as oats, barley, bulgur, and buckwheat; acorn and butternut squash; cooked peas, beans, and lentils; berries; and dried fruit and nuts.

▲ Look for whole-grain bread that contains 3 grams of fiber per serving and whole-grain crackers that contain at least 2 grams of fiber per serving.

▲ Baked products, such as muffins or cookies, can be prepared with whole-wheat flour. Any recipe calling for all-purpose flour may use 1/2 whole-wheat flour and 1/2 all-purpose flour. To use only whole-wheat flour, substitute 1 cup of whole-wheat flour minus 1 tablespoon for every 1 cup of all-purpose flour.

Fiber Content of Common Foods

CARBOHYDRATES (1 serving = 15 grams of carbohydrate)	Grams of Fiber
Cereals	
1/2-3/4 cup, low-fiber cereals ex. Cheerios, Wheaties, oatmeal	2-3
1/2-3/4 cup moderate fiber cereals ex. Bran Flakes, Shredded Wheat, oat bran	4-5
1/3-1/2 cup high fiber cereals ex. Fiber One, All-Bran, Fiber One	8-14
Breads/Crackers 1 serving whole grain or whole wheat	2
Grains 1/3 cup kasha, couscous, barley, bulgur, brown rice	2
Starchy Vegetables 1/2 cup corn, peas	3
Legumes 1/2 cup dried beans, peas and lentils	4-7
Fruit 1/2 cup or 1 small fruit	2-3
Vegetables 1/2 cup cooked 1-2 cups raw	2 3
Fat Nuts and seeds, 1/2 ounce	2-3

Ways to Add Fiber to Your Meals

▲ Eat fruits and vegetables with the skin or peel.

▲ Add low-fat granola to yogurt or fresh fruit.

▲ Eat whole grain cereal (at least 4 grams of fiber per serving) with fresh fruit for breakfast.

▲ Use whole grain breads and cereals. (WHOLE grain flour should be listed as the FIRST ingredient.)

▲ Eat popcorn, vegetables or high-fiber crackers for snacks.

▲ Eat the skin on baked potatoes and leave the skin on when making mashed potatoes.

▲ Eat brown rice instead of white rice, and whole wheat pasta instead of white pasta

▲ Eat whole fruits and vegetables instead of drinking juice.

▲ Substitute whole wheat or rye flour for part of the white flour when baking.

> **Fiber can help you lose weight by making you feel full which, in turn, means you eat less.**

▲ Include more beans in your meals: add to casseroles, chili, burritos, soups and salads.

Glycemic Index and Glycemic Load

Have you ever noticed that even though you carefully measure your carbohydrate servings or count your carbohydrate grams, you still can't always explain the level of your blood glucose after a meal? The glycemic index (GI) of foods may shed some light on this. Different foods may have the same number of carbs and yet not have the same effect on blood glucose. The glycemic index is a system of ranking foods containing equal amounts of carbohydrate according to how much they raise blood glucose levels. For instance, the carbohydrate in a slice of 100% stone-ground whole wheat bread (a low glycemic index food) may have less impact on your blood glucose than a slice of processed white bread (a high glycemic index food) even though both contain 15 grams of carb. The GI may be an additional meal-planning tool to help you understand how carbohydrate foods can differ in their effects on your blood glucose.

Researchers are in the process of measuring the GI of carbohydrate foods. Based on testing, foods are given a GI number that typically ranges from 0 to 100. Foods with lower numbers have less of an effect on blood glucose than do foods with higher numbers. Researchers determine the effect on blood glucose of a reference food, either 50 grams of glucose or 50 grams of bread, and then compare that effect to the effect of 50 grams of various other carbohydrate foods. The result of this comparison is expressed as a percentage. When using glucose — which has a GI of 100 — as a reference, a food is considered to be "low-GI" if its ranking falls between 0 and 55, "intermediate-GI" if it falls between 56 and 69, and "high-GI" if its ranking is 70 or greater. The methods by which GI is calculated are not always standard, so knowing the exact GI number is not as important as knowing in general if it is a low, moderate, or high GI food (that is, if the food has a low, moderate or high effect on blood glucose). The table on the following page lists examples of low, moderate, and high GI foods.

Examples of Low, Moderate and High Glycemic Index (GI) Foods

Low GI Foods	Moderate GI Foods	High GI Foods
Whole-grain breads	Rye bread	White bread
Bran cereals	Frosted Flakes	Corn Chex
Green grapes	Fruit cocktail	Watermelon
Cooked barley	Canned sweet corn	Instant mashed potatoes
Milk	Soft drinks	Sports drinks

Many factors affect how the carbohydrate in foods ranks on the GI scale. For example, highly processed foods, such as white bread, generally have higher GI values than foods that are not as processed. Fiber, protein, fat, and acidity all slow digestion and lower a food's GI value. Interestingly, sugars, fruit, and fruit juice usually have lower GI values as well. Sugars, either natural or added, are half glucose and half fructose. Fructose is primarily stored in the liver, so 50 grams of a sugar will raise blood glucose levels only about half as much as a similar portion of glucose. *If a food has a low GI, this does not mean that people with diabetes can eat unlimited amounts without it affecting their blood glucose levels.* Nor does it mean you have to eliminate all high GI foods, but rather try to combine them with low or moderate GI foods. Generally, when a high GI food is combined with a low GI food, the meal will be within the moderate GI range—for example, milk (low GI) with a cereal made primarily from corn (high GI) together will have a moderate GI.

The glycemic index can sometimes be difficult to apply to everyday eating situations because foods are compared to one another, not in usual portions, but in equal amounts of carbohydrate. For example, a pound and a half of carrots and one cup of spaghetti each have 50 grams of carbohydrate and this amount is used to determine their GI even though it is very unlikely anyone would consume that many carrots at one time!

Glycemic Load
Because of the challenge of relating GI to portion size, another approach can be used, called *glycemic load*. The glycemic load (GL) combines the GI value and the carbohydrate content of an average serving of a food, of a meal, or of a day's worth of food. The table on the next page lists some foods and their GI and GL.

Glycemic Index (GI) and Glycemic Load (GL) of Some Common Foods

Food	Serving Size	Grams of Carbohydrate	GI	GL
Pizza	1 slice	78	86	68
White rice	1 cup	45	102	46
Potatoes	1	37	102	38
Orange juice	6 oz.	20	75	15
White bread	1 slice	13	100	13
Carrots	1/2 cup	8	131	10
Milk	8 oz.	11	46	5

The glycemic load of a food is calculated by multiplying the GI number of the food by the actual number of grams of carbohydrate in a single serving and then dividing that number by 100:

GL = (GI x the number of carb grams per serving) divided by 100

A GL of 10 or less is low; 11-19 is medium; and 20 or more is high. Based on the chart above, carrots have a high GI (remember, the GI for carrots is arrived at by comparing 50 grams of carbs in carrots to 50 grams of carbs in the reference food – and it would take one and a half pounds of carrots to get 50 grams); therefore, you might think you need to avoid them. However, the GL (based on both the GI and the amount of carb in one serving of carrots) is only 10, which puts them in the low category.

Neither the glycemic index nor glycemic load should be used as the main method of meal planning for people with diabetes. The first step is to focus on the total amount of carbohydrate you eat. However, you may find that consistently choosing foods with a low GI and GL may help as you learn more about how certain foods improve your blood glucose levels.

NOTES

CHAPTER 7
Heart-Healthy Eating

....

People with diabetes are more likely to develop cardio-vascular complications (problems with the heart and blood vessels). These are the most common long-term problems that develop among those with diabetes. High blood glucose levels damage blood vessels. They make the walls thicker and less elastic so blood has a harder time passing through. Also, people with diabetes tend to have higher fat levels in their blood. High blood glucose levels can cause this. These fats or "lipids" clog and narrow the blood vessels. Sometimes they clog completely. These problems are referred to as atherosclerosis. Any blood vessel in your body can become narrow and clogged, and this can lead to a heart attack, angina (heart pain), stroke, or painful legs. There's no totally certain way to avoid heart disease and circulation problems. But there area number of things to do to cut your risk.

▲ If you smoke, stop.
▲ Lose weight if you are overweight
▲ Keep your blood pressure in the proper range
▲ Get regular physical activity
▲ Keep your blood fats and cholesterol levels in a healthy range
▲ Keep your blood glucose under control

> Controlling your cholesterol and blood pressure can lower your risk for cardiovascular complications!

Lipids (Blood Fats)

Fat and cholesterol are often mentioned together but they are not the same. Cholesterol is not a fat, but it does act together with fats in the body. Cholesterol is a waxy, fat-like substance made in your liver. Your body uses it to make bile and some hormones. If your body has too much cholesterol, it can be deposited on the walls of your arteries. This process results in the build-up of plaque, which can narrow blood vessels. Plaques can rupture and lead to blood clots, which in turn, can lead to a heart attack, stroke, or blockage in the blood vessels in the legs. To help reduce the build-up of these plaques, your total blood cholesterol should be 200 mg/dl or lower.

However, more important than your total cholesterol is the type of cholesterol made by your body — good or bad. LDL (which stands for low-density lipoprotein) cholesterol is considered "bad" because it can be deposited into the arteries. Your LDL cholesterol should be 100 mg/dl or lower. If you already have heart disease or are otherwise deemed to be at high risk (such as having diabetes), your healthcare provider may recommend that your LDL cholesterol be closer to 70 mg/dl. If your LDL level is above target, learn about ways to reduce your saturated fat, trans fat and cholesterol intake. In addition, your doctor may prescribe a medication to help lower your LDL level. If you do start on medication, remember that you must still continue to limit your intake of harmful fats and cholesterol.

On the other hand, HDL (high-density lipoprotein) cholesterol is considered "good" because it actually sweeps cholesterol from the arteries and carries it back to the liver, where it is reprocessed or eliminated. Ideally, men's HDL cholesterol should be above 40 mg/dl and women's above 50 mg/dl. If your HDL level is below target, try the following suggestions to help increase it:

▲ If you smoke, stop smoking!
▲ Aim to be physically active most days of the week, as activity can raise HDL levels.

▲ Use monounsaturated fats, such as olive or canola oil, for cooking and for adding to foods.

▲ Lose weight, if you need to.

While alcohol may actually help to raise HDL levels, it's not a generally recommended treatment. However, if you do drink alcohol, be sure to limit your servings to two per day (for men) or one per day (for women). Always discuss the use of alcohol with your healthcare provider. For more information about alcohol, see Chapter 11.

People with diabetes also need to be concerned with blood levels of *triglycerides*, a type of fat stored in fat cells as body fat, and burned for energy. High levels of triglycerides are linked with an increased risk of heart and blood vessel disease. Your triglyceride levels should be 150 mg/dl or lower. Keeping your blood glucose levels as near normal as possible can improve your triglyceride levels. Further, shedding a few extra pounds and doing regular physical activity can also be beneficial. Of course, being careful of your saturated fat and trans fat intake also helps improve triglycerides.

Lowering your risk of heart and blood vessel disease means reducing your intake of some types of food fats and food cholesterol, and substituting and using healthy food fats. Reducing your intake of sodium, losing some weight and doing regular physical activity will also lower your blood pressure.

Lipid Goals:

Total Cholesterol	200 mg/dl or lower
LDL	100 mg/dl or lower (70 mg/dl for some)
HDL	40 mg/dl or higher for men; 50 mg/dl or higher for women
Triglycerides	150 mg/dl or lower

The types and amounts of fat you eat and your sodium (salt) consumption play a major role in the development of heart disease and stroke. To reduce the risk of developing these problems, both you and your healthcare providers should pay close attention to your lipid (blood fat) and blood pressure numbers.

Food Fats

Fat is high in calories, so eating less fat can also help you control your weight. Fat packs a double punch of calories into every gram: A gram of fat contains nearly 9 calories, compared with only 4 calories for every gram of carbohydrate or protein. Extra pounds put a strain on your heart and also make your body's cells more resistant to insulin, which means that the insulin in your body doesn't work as well. Eating less fat, especially saturated fats, can help lower blood cholesterol and triglyceride levels. Changing the type of fat you eat can also help keep your heart and blood vessels healthy—not just for people with diabetes, but for everyone.

There are three types of food fat: *saturated fat* and *unsaturated fat* (both *polyunsaturated* and *monounsaturated*) and *trans fats*. Saturated fat is solid at room temperature. Foods that contain saturated fat include butter, shortening, fatty meats, whole milk, cheese, hydrogenated fats, and tropical oils. *Trans fat* is a type of fat formed from hydrogenation, a chemical process that changes a liquid oil into a solid fat. The process involves adding hydrogen to the unsaturated liquid oil and changing it into a saturated, solid fat. *Trans fats* are found in processed foods, such as snack foods, cookies, fast foods, and some stick or solid margarines. Both saturated fats and trans fats can raise cholesterol levels and should be eaten in as small amounts as possible.

Unsaturated fats come primarily from vegetables and are liquid at room temperature. *Polyunsaturated* fats include safflower, corn, sunflower and soybean oils, and fish, and can help lower cholesterol levels. Another important type of fat is omega-3 fatty acids. These are a type of polyunsaturated fats found in fish, flax seed and walnuts. This kind of fat can help lower triglyceride levels and lower the risk of heart disease. Monounsaturated fats include olive, canola and peanut oils, peanuts, olives, avocados, and nuts. Monounsaturated fats also help lower blood cholesterol levels and may help to raise HDL cholesterol levels.

Food Cholesterol

Cholesterol is often found in combination with fat in foods and acts similarly to saturated fats in the body. Cholesterol can be made in the liver or intestines, but is also found in some of the foods we eat. Cholesterol is found only in animal foods, such as eggs, milk, cheese, liver, meat and poultry. Eating too much cholesterol may increase your blood cholesterol levels. The goal is to limit your cholesterol intake to no more than 300 mg per day. If your LDL cholesterol is higher than 100 mg/dl, it may be helpful to lower your cholesterol intake to less than 200 mg per day. However, saturated fat and trans fat actually raise your blood cholesterol more than cholesterol found in food. Therefore, your first step in lowering your cholesterol level is to limit foods high in saturated fat and trans fat. And, the good news is that when you lower your intake of saturated fat (which is typically found in animal foods), you usually lower your intake of food cholesterol as well.

Plant Stanols and Sterols

You may have noticed margarine-like spreads that contain *plant stanol esters* (Benecol) or plant sterol esters (Take Control) in the supermarket and wondered if they really work. Plant stanol and sterol esters block the absorption of cholesterol in the intestine. Plant stanols are made from substances in plants that are combined with canola oil to form stanol esters, while plant sterols are made from soy. Both stanols and sterols can lower blood cholesterol levels. Research shows that eating about 2 grams (2 teaspoons) per day decreases total and LDL cholesterol by about 10%. They are not a drug and can be used safely in combination with cholesterol-lowering drugs such as statins. Stanols and sterols are found in other foods, as well, such as certain brands of orange juice (but keep in mind that 8 ounces of orange juice contains approximately 30 grams of carbohydrate!) and in some yogurts.

Soluble Fiber

Although not a fat, remember that eating foods containing soluble fiber can also lower blood cholesterol levels. Soluble fiber is a kind of fiber that can bind cholesterol in your intestines. Foods high in soluble fiber include oatmeal, oat bran, dried beans and peas, some fruits and vegetables, barley, and psyllium. For suggestions on how to increase fiber in your diet, see the previous section on fiber.

Tips to Reduce Your Intake of Saturated Fat and Cholesterol

Eating less saturated fat and cholesterol may help prevent and treat high blood cholesterol and triglyceride levels. An eating plan low in saturated fat can even help you prevent and treat high blood pressure. Below are some tips that will help:

▲ Use nonfat or low-fat dairy products, such as skim or 1% low-fat milk, nonfat or low-fat yogurt, and lower-fat cheeses.

▲ Limit your meal protein portions to 3 to 4 ounces. Most adults should limit total protein intake to about 6 ounces (after cooking) per day. Some women need only 4 to 5 ounces per day. People on meal plans of 2000 calories or more may be able to have up to 8 ounces of protein portions per day.

▲ Choose leaner cuts of meats, such as beef and pork tenderloin, and fish, and poultry (without skin). Look for luncheon meats with 3 grams or less of fat per ounce.

▲ Eat seafood, including fish and shellfish, often — at least two to three servings each week.

▲ Use olive, canola, or peanut oil for cooking instead of butter, lard, bacon fat or solid shortenings.

▲ Limit fatty snack foods, such as cookies, chips and some crackers.

▲ Cook using low-fat cooking methods such as baking, broiling, or roasting. When frying or sautéing foods, use a small amount of vegetable oil or a vegetable oil spray.

▲ Use a soft, tub margarine or one made with a plant stanol or sterol ester instead of butter, but be careful of amounts. The calories in margarine and butter are the same, but because butter is primarily a saturated fat, margarine is recommended. Look for margarine that lists a liquid oil such as corn, safflower, canola, or soybean as the first ingredient. A tub margarine is a better choice than solid or stick margarine. Better yet, look for a light (lower-fat and lower-calorie) tub margarine that is also trans fat free.

▲ Although not a fat, remember that eating foods containing soluble fiber can also lower blood cholesterol levels. Soluble fiber is a kind of fiber that can bind cholesterol in your intestines. Foods high in soluble fiber include oatmeal, oat bran, dried beans and peas, some fruits and vegetables, barley, and psyllium.

Sodium

A lower-sodium eating plan is important for preventing and treating high blood pressure (*hypertension*). Most of the sodium we eat comes from *sodium chloride* (table salt) added to processed foods or sprinkled on foods during preparation or eating. Sodium also occurs naturally in a wide variety of foods such as meats, dairy foods, and some vegetables.

Sodium is a mineral that is important for the body to function properly. For example, sodium helps regulate the fluid balance in your body and plays a role in maintaining blood pressure. However, most Americans eat far more sodium than they need. Research shows that sodium may contribute to some types of high blood pressure, a problem that many people with diabetes either have or are at greater risk of developing. In people with either normal or high blood pressure, reducing sodium intake lowers blood pressure. Because it is so important for people with diabetes to control blood pressure, daily intake of sodium should be limited to *less than 2300 milligrams (mg) per day* — that's equal to about a teaspoon of salt. By doing this, you may reduce your chances of high blood pressure and the risk of heart and blood vessel disease.

1/4 teaspoon salt	= 600 mg sodium
1/2 teaspoon salt	= 1200 mg sodium
3/4 teaspoon salt	= 1800 mg sodium
1 teaspoon salt	= 2400 mg sodium
1 teaspoon baking soda	= 1000 mg sodium

Tips for Reducing Sodium

Obvious ways to reduce sodium intake are to stop adding table salt to foods, and use minimal amounts of salt in cooking. There are salt substitutes that taste like salt but have little or no sodium. Some people find the taste is bitter, so try using a smaller amount than usual and experiment with different brands to find one you like. Although salt substitutes may be fine to use, you probably will do better cutting back on salt substitutes as well as salt. After a while, you will probably find you don't miss the taste. Some salt substitutes contain potassium chloride and people with kidney disease need to be careful about using products containing this mineral. If you have kidney disease, check with your healthcare provider before using a salt substitute.

The Nutrition Facts panel on food labels lists the amount of sodium in the serving size in milligrams. By definition, a low-sodium food is one that contains no more than 140 milligrams of sodium per serving. However, a good rule of thumb is to look for foods with 400 milligrams or less of sodium per serving, and 800 milligrams or less of sodium per convenience dinner or entrée.

Useful Definitions:

SODIUM FREE: 5 mg of sodium or less per serving

LOW SODIUM: 140 mg of sodium or less per serving

REDUCED SODIUM: At least 25% less sodium per serving as compared with a similar product

UNSALTED: Food product that is normally salted has been processed without salt

- ▲ Always taste your food before adding salt. Remove the saltshaker from the table.
- ▲ Eat fewer high-sodium smoked or cured meats such as bacon, hot dogs, and cold cuts. Instead, choose chicken, sliced turkey, and lean roast beef.
- ▲ Rely less on canned, packaged, and convenience foods. Rinsing canned foods with fresh water for about 30 seconds reduces their sodium content by one-half to three-fourths.
- ▲ Cook with less salt. Try herbs, spices, lemon juice, garlic, onion, and vinegar to flavor food. Substitute onion and garlic powders for onion and garlic salts.

▲ Limit high-sodium foods such as dill pickles, sauerkraut, chips, canned soups, and sauces such as ketchup, soy sauce, and steak sauce.

▲ Switch to low-sodium snacks. Instead of salted potato chips, salted nuts, and crackers, eat raw vegetables, fruits, and lower-salt crackers.

▲ Limit fast-foods, which tend to be higher in sodium than foods at sit-down restaurants.

▲ Remember that salt by any other name is still salt. Watch out for other high-sodium ingredients in foods, including baking soda, baking powder, sodium saccharin, seasoning salt, or any food that has sodium or salt in the name.

▲ Some over-the-counter medications are high in sodium, including Alka Seltzer, Bromo-Seltzer and some laxatives. Ask your healthcare provider about using these.

Instead of	Choose
Bacon, cold cuts, salt pork, corned/chipped beef, herring, sardines, smoked meats	Fresh/frozen beef, chicken, fish, veal, or other meats
Regular, hard and processed cheese	Low-sodium cheese
Regular peanut butter	Low-sodium peanut butter
Regular canned soup, soup mixes, broth, bouillon	Reduced-sodium canned soup, broth, bouillon
Canned vegetables, vegetable juice	Fresh/frozen vegetables or "no salt added" canned vegetables, lower sodium vegetable juice
Potato chips, pretzels, salted nuts, party dip and spread, crackers with salted tops	Unsalted pretzels, nuts, popcorn, crackers, mini rice cakes
Regular salad dressing	Oil and vinegar, low sodium salad dressings
Salt, soy sauce, steak sauce, Worcestershire sauce	Herbs, spices, Mrs. Dash, black pepper

CHAPTER 8
Tips For Cooking and Baking

....

L earning how to cook and bake healthy foods can help to keep your diabetes under control. It is also important to learn healthy ways of cooking and baking because it is easier to change the way you cook foods than it is to change the food choices you make. Not only will you be able to eat more of your favorite foods if you can learn to make them with less sugar and fat, but you can even use your own recipe books if you know how to make healthy changes and substitutions.

Change how you cook to save on calories and fat:

▲ Bake, broil, steam, poach, or grill foods instead of frying or cooking in fat.

▲ Use a paste of cornstarch or flour mixed with water instead of roux (melted butter and flour) to thicken sauces.

▲ Make stews or soups ahead of time; refrigerate, and skim off the hard fat that floats on top.

▲ When making casserole dishes, cook onions or other vegetables in the microwave or a nonstick pan, rather than sautéing them in butter or oil.

▲ Toast bread for hot sandwiches without adding butter or margarine.

▲ Stir-fry foods with a nonstick vegetable spray, or use a reduced-fat broth, instead of oil.

▲ If you do cook with oil, use heart-healthy oils, such as canola, olive and peanut oils. Use sparingly!

- ▲ Use lean cuts of meat (trimmed of fat), and poultry (without skin).
- ▲ Ground turkey breast is a good substitute for hamburger if it's at least 90% lean.
- ▲ Try a meatless meal at least one night each week, such as vegetarian chili.

Change how you bake:

- ▲ Use nonstick spray to coat muffin tins, cake pans, and cookie sheets.
- ▲ Bake low-fat, lower-sugar versions of sweets, such as banana bread, oatmeal raisin cookies, and muffins.
- ▲ Use a heart-healthy oil, such as canola oil, when baking.
- ▲ Decrease the sugar and fat in recipes by 1/3 to 1/2 of the amount specified. As a general rule, aim for less than 1 tablespoon of sugar per serving. If a recipe calls for more than that, try reducing the amount of sugar, or use a sugar substitute recommended for baking.
- ▲ Try recipes that use artificial sweeteners as part of their ingredients. However, don't completely replace sugar in recipes with artificial sweeteners because some sugar is needed to provide volume, texture and color. Try substituting half the sugar called for in a recipe with the equivalent amount of sweetener.
- ▲ Substitute sugar-free gelatin and pudding for regular gelatin and pudding in recipes that do not require baking.
- ▲ Try fruit-based fat "substitutes"or use applesauce in place of some or all of the fat in baked goods.
- ▲ Remember that you might need to experiment with substitutions in your recipes.

Substitute ingredients with less fat and calories:

Try...	Instead of...	Save Fat (grams)	Calories
1 cup skim milk	1 cup whole milk	8	60
1 cup evaporated skim milk (chill well before whipping)	1 cup whipping cream	89	630
1 cup low-fat or fat-free sour cream	1 cup sour cream	40	260
1 oz. light cream cheese	1 oz. cream cheese	5	30
1 cup light mayonnaise	1 cup mayonnaise	96	800
2 egg whites or 1/4 cup egg substitute	1 whole egg	5	40
1 Tbsp. light margarine	1 Tbsp. margarine	6	50
1/2 cup applesauce (in baked goods)	1/2 cup oil	109	910
1 tsp. butter-flavor sprinkles	1 Tbsp. butter	12	100
1 cup part-skim ricotta cheese	1 cup whole milk ricotta cheese	13	100
6 packets aspartame sweetener	1/4 cup sugar	0	170
6 packets saccharin sweetener	1/4 cup sugar	0	170
3 packets acesulfame-K sweetener	1/4 cup sugar	0	170
1/4 cup sucralose sweetener	1/4 cup sugar	0	170

Use less of an ingredient:

▲ Use smaller amounts of cheese by using strong-tasting cheeses (Romano, extra-sharp cheddar, blue cheese). You get more flavor with less cheese.

▲ Use less oil in muffins, pancakes, and waffles—1 tablespoon per cup of flour is usually enough.

▲ Use extra vegetables, dried beans, pasta, or rice and less meat in soups, casseroles, and stews.

▲ Use half as much salt in recipes.

Add flavor:

▲ Use more herbs and spices for flavor when you use less fat or sugar.

▲ Add spices, such as cinnamon and nutmeg, and vanilla or almond extracts to bring out the natural sweetness of foods.

▲ Season fresh vegetables with herbs and spices, herb vinegars, lemon juice, or soy sauce — try cinnamon on carrots, lemon juice on broccoli.

▲ Marinate meats before grilling or baking. Try tomato juice, soy sauce, sherry or wine, lemon juice, mustard, ginger, and other herbs and spices.

Enjoy a bit of the real thing:

▲ Some cookies, pies, and other desserts don't taste the same with less fat and sugar. Your dietitian can show you how to include the regular version of these foods in your meal plan.

▲ Make small batches of foods higher in fat or sugar and share them with friends.

▲ Try store-bought sugar-free or low-fat foods. However, be sure to read the label before you buy these foods. Some low-fat foods are high in carbohydrate. Also, some sugar-free foods are high in carbohydrate and fat.

CHAPTER 9
Supermarket Smarts

....

General Shopping Tips

▲ Using your meal plan, create a menu of at least one week's worth of meals and write them down on index cards or in a notebook where you can refer to them. Use the sample menus, starting on page 28, if you need ideas.

▲ Using your menus, write up a list of food items you'll need. Using a list will help limit the impulse to buy less healthy food. The list will also ensure that you have all the ingredients available when you prepare meals and snacks. Keep a master copy of your list to use whenever you shop.

▲ Read the weekly supermarket flyers in your area for specials on fruits, vegetables and other healthy foods.

▲ Use coupons only for items that you use and that are healthy. Resist the temptation to buy a high-fat ice cream, for example, just because you have a coupon.

▲ Grocery-shop after you've eaten a snack or a meal. Feeling hungry while you're shopping increases the chances that you'll buy high-fat, high-sugar foods.

▲ Select most of your foods from the outer aisles of the store, where most unprocessed foods are located. Be wary of featured food items at the end of the aisles; these foods tend to be higher in fat, sugar and calories.

▲ Read food labels to compare similar foods, such as cereals or crackers, focusing on serving size, total fat, total carbohydrate and fiber.

Healthy Food Choices

Grains, Beans & Starchy Vegetables (6-11 servings per day)	Milk & Dairy (3 servings per day)
• Whole-grain breads, bagels and cereals • Couscous, barley, bulgur • White, brown or wild rice, pasta • Dried beans (pinto, kidney, split pea, blackeyed peas, lentils) • Corn, green peas, potato or winter squash	• Skim or low-fat (1%) milk • Low-fat or fat-free yogurt, plain or sweetened with artificial sweetener • Reduced-fat or fat-free American, mozzarella, cheddar, or cottage cheese (3 grams fat or less per serving)
Meat & Meat Substitutes (up to 6 ounces per day)	**Fruits & Vegetables** (2 cups fruits, 2-1/2 or more cups vegetables per day)
• Chicken and turkey (skin removed) • Fresh or frozen fish (cod, tuna, haddock), without breading; lean beef (round, sirloin, flank) • Lean pork (tenderloin or center-cut) • Fat-free hot dogs • Egg whites or egg substitutes • Light tofu	• Fresh, frozen, or canned vegetables without sauces added • Fresh, dried or canned fruit packed in juice • Fruit juices, without added sweeteners or syrups
Snack Foods (in limited quantities)	**Fats & Oils** (in limited quantities)
• Low-fat crackers • Low-fat popcorn • Baked chips or pretzels • Rice cakes • Low-fat cookies: vanilla wafers, gingersnaps, graham crackers, animal crackers • Sugar-free pudding or gelatin	• Canola, olive, or peanut oil • Soft tub margarine (trans fatty acid free) • Nonfat or light sour cream • Fat-free or low-fat mayonnaise and salad dressings • Fat-free or low-fat cream cheese • Peanut butter

CHAPTER 10
Eating Out with Diabetes

···

One of the most enjoyable aspects of eating out has absolutely nothing to do with food; rather, it's the pleasure of spending time with family, friends and colleagues. By focusing on the social element of the dining-out experience, you will develop a healthier mind-set. Part of this mind-set is to adapt to the unexpected — food that isn't prepared right, slow service, or the temptation to eat foods you know you probably shouldn't. If the unexpected happens, your meal will still be enjoyable because you have already decided that the most important part of eating out is to enjoy the company of your friends and family. And people with diabetes can and should enjoy dining out just as much as people who don't have diabetes.

Eating out doesn't just mean going to a restaurant to eat a meal. It can mean a drive-up window at a fast-food restaurant, eating at a ballpark, food court, or during an after-work meeting. Or it can be food you purchase at a deli or restaurant and take home to eat, such as a chicken dinner, pizza, or Chinese food. Unfortunately, the foods that are available away from home are usually higher in total and saturated fat, cholesterol, sodium, and sugars. And whole grains, fruits, and vegetables are often not available.

Of course, eating healthy foods should still remain high on your list. Even though you are away from your own kitchen, you can and should still control what you eat. By adapting guidelines you've learned for managing your diabetes at home, you can develop a strategy for eating out. Following are a few strategies that may help you enjoy both your food choices and your friends and family.

▲ Know your meal plan and the number of carbohydrate servings you have at meals. When eating out, try and stay with your meal plan as much as possible, especially your number of carbohydrate servings.

▲ Choose a restaurant carefully. Look for restaurants that offer a wide selection of broiled and baked foods, such as fish and poultry. Avoid restaurants that offer only large portions of fatty meats and fried foods, like large prime steaks, fried chicken or fish. Call the restaurant ahead of time to ask about the menu, or go on the Internet— many restaurants now post their menus online.

▲ Plan ahead for what you will order. It's helpful if you are familiar with the menu offerings and preplan what you might order before even seeing the menu. Try to be the first to order so you're not tempted to change your mind when you hear what your friends are ordering. Choose dishes that are grilled, baked, broiled, poached, steamed, roasted or lightly sautéed. Most restaurants will allow you to customize your order to make your meal more nutri tious. See the table below, *Healthy Choices for Dining Out*, for other menu suggestions.

▲ Be aware of the "dangers" from all-you-can-eat restaurants. You many think an all-you-can-eat buffet is a good option. After all, you will be able to see the food, determine how it is prepared, and serve your own portions. If you have fantastic self-control, this strategy may work. But remember, these places are billed as "all-you-can-eat," not "all-you-should-eat." Too often you may be tempted to pile far too much food on your plate, especially if the food all looks so good that it's hard to resist. Salad bars pose a similar temptation. If you stick to fresh vegetables and low-calorie dressings, you'll do fine. But watch out for all the other prepared salads, cheese, eggs, gelatins, and high-fat salad dressings.

▲ **Count your carbs carefully!** Foods high in carbohydrate are abundant at restaurants, from the bread basket on the table to the rice piled high on your plate. Watch your portions. If you crave the hot, homemade rolls, ask if you can have a non-starchy vegetable in place of the rice or potato in your entrée.

▲ **Ask for sauces and dressings on the side.** By controlling how much salad dressing you put on your salad, or gravy on your meat, you'll end up using less and will decrease your fat and calorie intake.

▲ **Eyeball the portions.** Large portions are a fact of restaurant dining. Practicing portion control at home (weighing and measuring your foods periodically) will help you control portions when you're away from home. And don't forget the system restaurants have long used to help you with portion control — the doggie bag! Ask your server to package up half your meal in the kitchen before it's served to you, or ask your server to bring a take-home container to your table when your meal is served; before you dig in, put half of your meal in the container.

▲ **Look out for "supersize" terms.** Watch out for fast food terms such as jumbo, extra-large, deluxe or supersized. Go with regular or junior-sized items instead to save calories, fat and sodium.

▲ **Share an entrée with your dining companion or order off the appetizer menu (as long as the choices are healthy).** Many restaurant entrées are large enough for two people, so see if your family member or friend will split a meal with you. Some restaurants will offer half portions of entrées as well.

▲ **Make requests.** Restaurants are in the business to "serve" people and usually try to comply with reasonable requests that are asked in a pleasant and non-threatening manner. For example, you might try asking for your fish to be broiled with olive oil instead of butter.

▲ Look up nutrition information for chain or fast food restaurants before leaving home. Many of these restaurants post their information on the Internet. There are also many food count books that compile the information for you.

▲ Be realistic. Accept the fact that nobody is perfect all the time. Whether you are eating at home or away, do the best you can. And if you have a momentary lapse, keep it a momentary lapse. Just pick up where you left off and continue your diabetes management with a positive out look. If you've overeaten, don't feel guilty, but instead go for a walk or do some other physical activity after the meal to help lower your blood glucose and burn off calories.

▲ Consider eating a small snack if your meal will be later than usual. If you prefer to take your diabetes pills before you leave for the restaurant, and you expect your meal to be later, you may need to eat a small snack to "hold you over" and prevent the possibility of a low blood glucose. Your healthcare team can give you guidance on the timing of your medications and your meals.

▲ And finally, if you take a rapid-acting insulin before meals, learn how to adjust your dose to appropriately cover the carbohydrate you eat. If you're using your insulin-to-carbohydrate ratio (see Advanced Carbohydrate Counting, page 21) to make adjustments based on the number of carbohydrate servings you plan to eat. You can take your insulin (and diabetes pills) after you get to the restaurant or even, for rapid-acting insulin, when the food is being brought to the table in case your meal is served late. Check your blood glucose more often whenever you eat meals at different times.

> Dessert isn't necessarily off limits; split a dessert with your spouse or friend – just make sure to count your carbs!

Healthy Choices for Dining Out

Breakfast: cereal with skim or 1% low-fat milk; whole-grain toast, bagels, English muffins; boiled or poached eggs; omelets made with egg substitutes; pancakes or waffles with fruit; Canadian bacon

Appetizers: shrimp or crab cocktail; chicken teriyaki; raw vegetables; fresh fruit cup; bouillon or consommé; broth-based soups

Fast Foods: regular or junior-sized burgers without cheese and sauces; grilled chicken sandwiches; small fries; salads with low-calorie dressings

Pizza: thin-crust pizza with vegetable toppings; "cheese-less" pizzas

Delis: sandwiches made with turkey or chicken breast, lean roast beef, lean ham; vegetables, hummus; mustard instead of mayonnaise

Mexican: fajitas, burritos or soft tacos with chicken or bean fillings; Mexican rice, black beans on the side; salsa, chopped vegetables

Italian: minestrone, pasta fagioli soup; plain Italian bread; pasta with chicken or seafood in a vegetable, marinara (tomato) or light wine sauce

Chinese: wonton, hot-and-sour soup; stir-fried vegetables with meat, seafood or poultry (not deep-fried); mu-shu dishes; vegetarian dishes; steamed vegetables and brown rice

American: broiled, grilled or stir-fried poultry, seafood, and lean meat dishes; baked or boiled potatoes, brown or wild rice; steamed or lightly sautéed vegetables (without added butter)

NOTES

CHAPTER 11
Alcohol

··

Alcoholic beverages are a common part of many peoples' social lives. If you drink alcohol you should understand what the potential effects of alcohol are on your diabetes control. Perhaps you are someone who has routinely enjoyed having an occasional drink on social occasions or a glass of wine with dinner. Now that you have diabetes, you may wonder if you should continue doing this.

Alcohol guidelines for adults with diabetes are similar to those for the general public: men should limit alcoholic drinks to two or less per day and women one or less per day. One drink contains about 15 grams of alcohol and is defined as a:

▲ 12-oz. beer (preferably light)

▲ 5-oz. glass of wine

▲ 1-1/2 oz. distilled spirits ("hard liquor," such as scotch, whiskey, or vodka)

If you drink alcohol in moderation and with food, it will have minimal, if any, effect on your blood glucose or insulin levels. However, if you take insulin or some of the diabetes pills, and if alcohol is consumed without food, alcohol can lower blood glucose, causing low blood glucose reactions. Alcohol is absorbed directly from the stomach into the bloodstream and carried to the liver, where it is broken down (metabolized). While the liver is processing alcohol, its ability to release glucose is blocked. In other words, the liver is "distracted" from doing its regular job. This can cause blood glucose levels to drop, especially if no food is eaten, and the result is the risk, for up to 10 to 12 hours after drinking, of a low blood glucose reaction.

To lower the chances of having a low blood glucose, you should follow your usual meal plan when drinking an alcoholic beverage. No food should be omitted. Food in the stomach also slows down the absorption of alcohol into the bloodstream and lowers the amount of alcohol that reaches the liver at one time. The liver can perform better while processing smaller amounts of alcohol. In addition, if you drink alcohol in the evening, be sure to check your blood glucose before you go to sleep. You may need to eat a snack to prevent your blood glucose from dropping during the night. Also, be aware that if you exercise and drink alcohol (for example, having a few beers after playing a game of basketball), your risk of having a low blood glucose later on increases, as well. For this reason, it's important to monitor your blood glucose levels more often whenever you drink alcohol.

> **Drink your alcohol with your meal to lessen the chance of having a low blood glucose.**

As a general guideline, two alcoholic beverages may be an occasional addition to your regular meal plan. Again, no food should be omitted in exchange for an alcoholic drink. Because 12 ounces of regular beer contains about 14 grams of carbohydrate, a light beer may be a better choice. Some alcoholic beverages contain higher amounts of sugar, such as wine coolers and liqueurs. Use these sparingly as they may increase your blood glucose levels. Twelve ounces of nonalcoholic beer also contain about 15 grams of carbohydrate and should be counted as one carbohydrate choice in your meal. If you're trying to lose weight, remember that alcohol contributes calories even if it doesn't affect blood glucose. For example, one 12-oz light beer, a 5-oz. glass of wine, or a 1-1/2 oz. "shot" of hard liquor are each about 100 calories. In fact, alcohol contains 7 calories per gram, almost as much as fat, which contains 9 calories per gram. The table, *Alcoholic Beverages*, on page 85 lists the calories and grams of carbohydrate in common alcoholic beverages.

Some people with diabetes should not drink, including pregnant and lactating women, and people with medical problems such as pancreatitis, advanced neuropathy (diabetic nerve disease), or a history of alcohol abuse. Incidentally, recent research has also shown that moderate amounts of alcohol do not raise triglyceride levels, but should be avoided if triglyceride levels are extremely high. Excessive amounts of alcohol may increase blood pressure and may also worsen retinopathy (diabetic eye disease). Finally, if you take metformin to help control your diabetes, do not drink large amounts of alcohol. Doing so may increase your risk of developing lactic acidosis, a rare but serious metabolic complication.

There may be beneficial effects from drinking small to moderate amounts of alcohol. For example, in adults with type 2 diabetes, one to two drinks per day is linked with a lower risk of heart disease and increased insulin sensitivity. However, the research is not strong enough to recommend that adults who don't drink now should start. Alcohol appears to increase HDL (the "good") cholesterol, which has a protective effect against heart disease. But regular exercise can have the same effect and for many adults will be more appropriate.

Guidelines for Alcohol

The message is always the same. Avoid large intakes of alcoholic beverages. However if you choose to occasionally have a "drink," the following guidelines can help you safely enjoy the occasion:

▲ Drink alcoholic beverages along with food. This is especially important if you use insulin or take diabetes pills. Signs and symptoms of a low blood glucose and intoxication are similar and your companions may just think you are a little "tipsy" instead of hypoglycemic. Make sure your friends know you have diabetes and know how to treat a low blood glucose.

▲ For men, limit the amount to 2 drinks or less per day, and for women 1 drink or less per day. A drink is defined as a 12-ounce beer (preferably light beer), a 5-ounce glass of wine, or 1-1/2 ounces of a distilled beverage, such as whiskey, rum, vodka or gin.

▲ Limit alcohol if you are trying to lose weight. Even if it doesn't affect your blood glucose, alcohol can still contribute significant calories.

▲ Mix hard liquor such as gin, rum, whiskey, bourbon, scotch and vodka with water or sugar-free beverages rather than juices, regular sodas or regular tonic water which add calories and carbohydrate.

▲ Check with your healthcare providers to see if you are taking other medications that might interact with alcohol, or if there are other reasons you should avoid alcoholic beverages.

▲ Drink safely and smartly. Carry or wear identification that states that you have diabetes.

▲ Follow all precautions that are encouraged for all adults — drink in moderation and don't drink and drive.

Alcoholic Beverages — Calories and Carbs

Beverage	Amount	Calories	Carbohydrate grams (g)
Beer			
Regular beer	12 ounces	150	14
Light beer	12 ounces	100	5
Non-alcoholic beer	12 ounces	70	15
Distilled spirits			
Gin, rum, vodka, whiskey, scotch, bourbon	1.5 ounces	105	Trace
Wine			
Red or rosé	5 ounces	105	3
White	5 ounces	100	1
Sweet wine	2 ounces	90	7
Wine coolers	12 ounces	190	22
Champagne	4 ounces	100	4
Vermouth	3 ounces	105	4
Cocktails			
Gin & tonic	7.5 ounces	225	16
Martini	2.5 ounces	160	0
Daiquiri	4 ounces	220	2
Bloody Mary	5 ounces	115	5
Liqueurs/cordials	1.5 ounces	160	18

NOTES

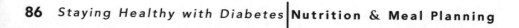

CHAPTER 12
Holidays and Special Occasions

··

Holidays are special occasions for all of us, and on such occasions, some flexibility with meal planning is needed. If you take insulin and adjust your insulin doses based on your carbohydrate intake, being flexible is fairly easy. Even if you don't make such adjustments, straying from your meal plan will not affect your long-term health as long as you get back on track the next day.

Vacations can also be challenging, as eating variations are not focused on one day but over a week or more. While the excess seen on Thanksgiving or one's birthday is not recommended for a week's vacation, it's likely that following your meal plan exactly just won't be realistic or possible. Try to limit the excursions from the meal plan to foods that are "worth it" such as a special dinner, but try to keep on target for breakfast and lunch. Certainly, when you're back home, making a strong effort to get back on track immediately is important. Here are some other tips to help get you through the holidays and special occasions:

▲ Plan ahead. Think about the types of foods that may be served at Thanksgiving dinner or a holiday party, and decide what you'll have before you start eating. If you want a piece of pumpkin pie, for example, determine how many grams of carb is in the pie, and substitute it for another carb food at your meal (or adjust your insulin dose accordingly). Offer to bring a dish to a party that you feel comfortable eating.

▲ Try to eat at your regular meal times as much as possible. If your meal is delayed, eat a small snack at your regular meal time.

▲ Monitor your blood glucose levels more often than usual to help you stay in better control.

▲ Try not to linger at the buffet table at parties.

▲ Limit your intake of alcohol; if you do drink, be sure to eat some food with your cocktail.

▲ Be as active as possible! Rather than taking a nap after a huge holiday meal, go out for a walk. Regular activity is important any time of the year, but is especially important on special occasions and vacations.

▲ Ask your dietitian for help. For example, he or she can help you figure out how to fit favorite foods into your meal plan, determine how many carbs are in certain seasonal or holiday foods, and how to alter recipes to make them more healthful.

CHAPTER 13
Meal Replacements

....

Meal replacements have become an integral part of today's busy lifestyle. More and more people use meal replacements for one or more meals or snacks throughout the day. Liquid supplements, bars and even frozen meals are all forms of meal replacements.

Many people drink a shake or eat a bar in place of a meal as part of a weight control plan. In fact, Joslin's Nutrition Guideline recognizes that meal replacements (shakes, bars and ready-to-mix powders) can be helpful for some people trying to lose weight. Others find it convenient to grab a shake in place of breakfast or as a light supper if they're on the go. Some people even use meal replacements as a supplement to their regular eating plan if, for example, they are trying to gain weight, or need extra nutrition while they recover from an illness or surgery. If you're thinking of trying a meal replacement, keep in mind the following guidelines:

▲ Don't use meal replacements for more than two meals per day, unless you're under the guidance of your healthcare provider.

▲ Some meal replacements, such as energy or nutrition bars, are no different than a candy bar. Read the nutrition labels carefully.

▲ Choose products with:
   • No more than 200-250 calories per serving
   • Approximately 5-10 grams of fat per serving
   • Approximately 3-5 grams of fiber per serving
   • Approximately 10-15 grams of protein per serving
   • One third of the recommended daily amount of vitamins and minerals

▲ Remember that shakes and bars should be used in place of a meal or snack — not in addition!

▲ Avoid supplements that only contain protein (often recommended for body builders) and do not contain carbohydrate, unless they've been suggested by your healthcare provider.

Finally, there are many specialty types of supplements (usually liquids or bars) on the market. Some, for example, contain slowly digested carbohydrate and fiber, and are geared for people with diabetes. Others may contain a blend of heart-healthy fats for people with high cholesterol levels or heart disease. These kinds of supplements may be fine for you to use, but always check with a dietitian before you begin using them to make sure they're appropriate. Your dietitian can also help you fit these into your meal plan.

CHAPTER 14
Eating on "Sick Days"

....

t is important that you continue to eat and drink on days when you are ill or just not feeling well. If you can't follow your meal plan but can still eat some food, choose items from the list below. Each item contains about 15 grams of carbohydrate (1 carb choice). Try to eat or drink 50 grams of carbohydrate (3 carb choices) every three to four hours. These are examples of foods that contain 15 grams of carbohydrate:

1/2 cup applesauce
1/2 cup apple juice
1/3 cup grape juice
1/3 cup fruited yogurt
1/2 cup regular Jello
1/4 cup milkshake
1 cup Gatorade
1 tablespoon honey
1/4 cup regular pudding
1 pop of a twin pop Popsicle
1/2 cup regular or light ice cream
1/2 cup eggnog
1/2 cup cooked cereal

Other food choices that you might try include salty foods like broth, consommé, and tomato juice; or soft solids like toast, hot cereals or soups. Eating foods that contain salt can help replace any sodium lost from gastrointestinal illness. If you feel too sick to eat, drink 6-8 ounces of liquid every hour. If you are unable to eat solid foods, you should switch back and forth between drinks that have carbohydrate in them, such as regular soft drinks and juice, one hour, and drinks that do not contain sugar, such as diet soft drinks, tea and water, for the next hour. Call your healthcare provider if you cannot keep anything down.

NOTES

CHAPTER 15
Vitamins, Minerals and Supplements

···

Vitamins and Minerals

Vitamins and minerals such as calcium, iron, potassium and zinc, are essential nutrients that are present — but only in small amounts — in the foods we eat. They are very important because they help the body process foods and are involved in many other body functions, including the metabolism of carbohydrate.

People with diabetes often ask if they should take vitamin or mineral supplements (capsules or tablets) available from drugstores or health food stores. If you are eating a balanced diet you may not need to take these supplements. But, since many people find it challenging to eat a balanced diet on a daily basis, it may be wise to consider taking a multivitamin/mineral supplement. Other people who may benefit from taking a multivitamin and mineral supplement include elderly persons, pregnant or lactating women, strict vegetarians, and individuals on calorie-restricted diets. And newer research has shown that people with type 2 diabetes who take a multivitamin/mineral supplement are less prone to developing infections. If you choose to take a multivitamin supplement, look for one that does not have more than approximately 100% of the Recommended Dietary Allowance (RDA) for any of the vitamins or minerals in it. Your dietitian can assist you in choosing a supplement that best fits your needs.

There are some people who may benefit from a specific supplement. All women of childbearing age need enough folic acid (a B vitamin) for the prevention of birth defects. And anyone not drinking milk is likely to have an inadequate calcium intake —

important for the prevention of bone disease—unless they take a calcium supplement. This may be especially important for women with type 1 diabetes who are at greater risk for developing osteoporosis. Pre-menopausal women may need extra iron. However, discuss the use of iron supplements with your healthcare provider before you start taking them. Older adults are at risk for specific nutrient deficiencies, such as vitamin B12 and vitamin D. If you are an older adult, speak with your healthcare provider or dietitian to learn if you should take specific supplements.

At the present time there are no vitamin, mineral, or other supplements that have a proven benefit for controlling blood glucose levels. While some supplements, such as chromium or ginseng, may have an effect on blood glucose levels, not enough is known about their action, safety and appropriate dosage to recommend their use for people with diabetes.

Although several small studies suggested that antioxidants—vitamin E, beta-carotene, vitamin C, and selenium—might protect against heart and vessel disease, large randomized trials involving over 81,000 persons in whom antioxidants were compared to placebos (fake antioxidants) found no benefit from the antioxidants in preventing heart and vessel disease in the general public or in people with diabetes. Of concern also are recent studies reporting that antioxidants hampered the beneficial effects of a statin (medication for cholesterol) and niacin on blood cholesterol values—they appear to prevent the increase in HDL (the "good") cholesterol usually seen from these medications. The American Diabetes Association nutrition recommendations have concluded that routine supplementation with antioxidants is not advised because of the uncertainties relating to long-term benefit and safety. What is important for the prevention of heart and vessel disease are lifestyle factors (nutrition and physical activity), aspirin, medications for lowering cholesterol and blood pressure, and smoking cessation. The jury is still out as to whether antioxidants can help prevent certain diseases and conditions, such as heart disease, stroke or some types of cancer. Be sure to talk with your dietitian or other healthcare provider if you are wondering about taking a supplement. They can help you decide what type and amount would be most likely to be beneficial for you.

Herbal and Other Dietary Supplements

There are a variety of herbal and botanical supplements that in animal studies or in small or poorly conducted studies in humans have been shown to improve glucose levels. However, in persons with diabetes there is little evidence to suggest benefit from any of the herbal supplements. What minimal evidence there is looks at substances such as cinnamon, which may improve blood glucose and lipid levels in people with type 2 diabetes, and there is also some research looking at alpha lipoic acid showing that this antioxidant may help reduce the frequency and severity of symptoms of diabetic neuropathy. However, be careful when using some of these herbs, botanicals and nutritional supplements as they may have the potential to interfere with medications you may be taking. These supplements may also affect your blood glucose levels, as well. Therefore, it is important that you discuss with your dietitian and healthcare provider any supplements you are taking or plan to take. And never substitute a supplement for a prescription drug without first checking with your healthcare providers.

> **These herbal supplements can be harmful, so avoid taking them:**
>
> aristolochic acid
> chaparral
> comfrey
> ephedra
> kava
> tiratricol
> usnic acid

NOTES

CHAPTER 16
Meal Planning — Simple!

To sum up, here are a few general points to keep in mind when thinking about meal planning and diabetes:

▲ Eat at about the same time each day.
▲ Eat about the same amounts of food each day and don't overeat.
▲ Eat a wide variety of foods each day.
▲ Use less added fat, sugar and salt.
▲ If you are overweight, cut down on portion sizes and fats to lose weight.

Eating healthfully, maintaining a realistic body weight and being physically active are all important ways to manage your diabetes. Your healthcare team is your partner in making sure that you stay as healthy as possible with diabetes. Periodically, your medical and nutritional goals may change. You may no longer need to lose weight, you may start a new exercise program, or you may move from oral medications to insulin to manage your diabetes, for example. In such cases, you will want to consult your dietitian yearly to update your meal plan or check your progress.

Before long, much of what is contained in this book will become second nature to you, and you will be ready to take the next steps toward more creative eating. For more information on all aspects of diabetes and diabetes management, refer to *The Joslin Guide to Diabetes*. Happy eating!

Joslin Food Lists

The following food lists, which are similar to the American Diabetes Association and American Dietetic Association's lists, will help you plan healthy meals and snacks. Use these lists as a guide, making sure that you aim for a balance of carbohydrate, protein and fat everyday. Be sure to take note of the portion size for one serving of a particular food, and remember that if you eat twice as much, you'll get twice as many calories and nutrients.

Food companies frequently change their products, which means that your best source of nutrition information is most always going to be the food's nutrition label. However, because many foods, such as fruits and vegetables, do not come with a label, the food lists can help ensure that you eat the right amount to help manage your blood glucose levels and your weight.

Carbohydrates List

A carbohydrate serving (approximately 15 grams) may include a food choice from the fruit, milk or starch categories. Vegetables are also carbohydrates, but contain fewer grams of carbohydrates (5 grams) per serving, so if you are using carbohydrate counting as your meal planning option, be sure to note the difference.

Starch Choices

BREADS

ITEM	SERVING SIZE
White, whole-wheat, rye, etc.	1 slice (1 oz.)
Raisin	1 slice (1 oz.)
Italian and French	1 slice (1 oz.)
"Light"	
(1 slice equals 40 calories)	2 slices
Pita	
pocket, 6 in. diameter	1/2 pocket
mini size	1 pocket
Bagel	1/4 large (1 oz.)
English muffin	1/2 small
Rolls	
bulkie	1/2 small
dinner, plain	1 small
frankfurter	1/2 medium
hamburger	1/2 medium
Bread Crumbs	3 Tbsp.
Croutons	3 Tbsp.
Taco Shells, small	2 (+1 Fat)
Tortilla, corn, 6 in. diameter	1
Tortilla, flour, 7 in. diameter	1 (+1 Fat)

BEST CHOICES: Whole grain breads and cereals, dried beans and peas.

One choice provides:
Calories: 80
Carb: 15 gms
Protein: 3 gms
Fat: 0-5 gms fat

CEREALS

ITEM	SERVING SIZE
Cooked cereals	1/2 cup
Bran:	
*All Bran with Extra Fiber	1/3 cup
*All Bran	1/3 cup
*Bran Flakes	1/2 cup
*Complete Wheat Bran Flakes	1/2 cup
*Fiber One	1/3 cup
Multibran Chex	1/3 cup
Cheerios	2/3 cup
Cheerios, Honey Nut	2/3 cup
Corn Chex	1/2 cup
Cornflakes	1/2 cup
Crispix	1/2 cup
Go Lean Crunch	1/2 cup
Good Friends	1/3 cup
Grapenuts	3 Tbsp.
*Grapenuts Flakes	1/3 cup
Just Right (with nuggets)	1/3 cup
Kix	3/4 cup
Life	1/2 cup
Product 19	2/3 cup
Puffed Kashi	1 cup
Puffed Rice, Wheat	1 cup
Raisin Bran	1/3 cup
Rice Krispies	2/3 cup
*Shredded Wheat biscuit	1 biscuit
*Shredded Wheat n' Bran	1/2 cup
Special K	3/4 cup
Total	1/2 cup
*Wheat Chex	1/3 cup
*Wheaties	2/3 cup

*Cereals high in fiber

STARCHY VEGETABLES

ITEM	SERVING SIZE
Corn	1/2 cup
Corn on the cob	1/2 cob
Mixed vegetables, with corn or peas	1 cup
Parsnips	1/2 cup
Peas, green, canned or frozen	1/2 cup
Plantain, cooked	1/2 cup
Potato, white	
mashed	1/2 cup
baked	1/4 large or 1 small (3 oz.)
Potato, sweet	
mashed	1/2 cup
baked	1 small or 1/2 cup (2 oz.)
Pumpkin	1 cup
Winter squash, acorn or butternut	1 cup

PASTA

Macaroni, noodles, spaghetti (cooked)	1/3 cup

LEGUMES

Beans, peas, lentils (cooked)	1/2 cup
Baked beans, canned, no pork (vegetarian style)	1/3 cup
Lima beans	2/3 cup
Miso	3 Tbsp.

GRAINS

ITEM	SERVING SIZE
Barley, cooked	1/3 cup
Bulgur, cooked	1/2 cup
Cornmeal	3 Tbsp.
Cornstarch	2 Tbsp.
Couscous, cooked	1/3 cup
Flour	3 Tbsp.
Kasha, cooked	1/2 cup
Millet, cooked	1/4 cup
Oats, cooked	1/2 cup
Quinoa, cooked	1/2 cup
Rice, cooked	1/3 cup
Wheat berries	2/3 cup
Wheat germ	1/4 cup
Wild rice	1/2 cup

COOKIES

ITEM	SERVING SIZE
Ak-Mak	10 (1 oz.)
Animal crackers	8
Arrowroots	5
Cheese Nips, reduced fat	22
Cheez-Its, reduced fat	22
Finn Crisp, original	2
Fig Newtons	2
Gingersnaps	3
*Goldfish pretzels	29
Graham crackers,	
2-1/2 in. squares	3
Granola bar, low-fat plain	1
Matzoh	1/2 board
Melba toast	4 slices
Nilla Wafers, reduced fat	5
Oyster crackers	24
Popcorn, microwave, light	4 cups
Popcorn: popped,	3 cups
no fat added	
*Pretzels	3/4 oz.
Rice cakes, popcorn cakes	2
Mini rice cakes	8
Rye Krisp, triple crackers	3
*Saltines	6
Social Teas	5

High in sodium

> **BEST CHOICES:** Low in saturated fat and sodium

CRACKERS

ITEM	SERVING SIZE
*Snack chips:	
Baked potato/tortilla chips	15-20 (3/4 oz.)
Stella D'Oro Anisette Toast	2
Stella D'Oro breadsticks	2
Stoned Wheat Thins	3
Stoned Wheat Thins, Mini	14
Teddy Grahams	16
Triscuits, reduced fat	5
Uneedas	4
WASA Extra Crisp; Light Rye	3
Water cracker	4
Wheat Thins, reduced fat	13
Zwieback toast	3

*High in sodium

FRUIT

BE SURE:
To choose fresh, frozen or canned fruit packed in its own juice or water with no added sugar. Eat at least 2 cups of fruit each day.

ITEM	SERVING SIZE
Apple, 4 oz.	1 small
Apple, dried	4 rings
Applesauce, unsweetened	1/2 cup
Apricots	
fresh	4 medium
canned	1/2 cup
dried	8 halves
Banana, 4 oz.	1/2
Blackberries	3/4 cup
Blueberries	3/4 cup
Canned fruit,	
unless otherwise stated	1/2 cup
Cantaloupe, 11 oz.	
sectioned	1/3
melon cubed	1 cup
Casaba, 7 in. diameter	
sectioned	1/6 melon
cubed	1-1/3 cups
Cherries, sweet fresh	12
Clementines	2
Dates	3
Figs, fresh	2 small
dried	1-1/2
Fruit Cocktail	1/2 cup
Granadilla (passion fruit)	4
Grapefruit, large	1/2
Grapes	17 small

> **BEST CHOICES:**
> Fresh fruit
>
> **One choice provides:**
> Calories: 60
> Carb: 15 gms
> Protein: 0 gms
> Fat: 0 gms

FRUIT (continued)

ITEM	SERVING SIZE
Guava	1 small
Honeydew melon, 10 oz.	
sectioned	1/8 melon
cubed	1 cup
Kiwi, 3 oz.	1 large
Kumquat	5 medium
Loquats, fresh	12
Lychees, fresh or dried	10
Mandarin oranges, canned	3/4 cup
Mango	1/2 small
sliced	1/2 cup
Nectarine, 5 oz.	1 small
Orange, 6-1/2 oz.	1 small
Papaya, 8 oz.	
sectioned	1/2
cubed	1 cup
Peach, 4 oz.	1 medium
Pear, 4 oz.	1/2 large
Persimmon	2
Pineapple,	
fresh, diced	3/4 cup
canned	1/2 cup
Plum, 5 oz.	2 small
Pomegranate, 5 oz.	1/2
Prunes, dried	3 medium
Raisins	2 Tbsp.
Raspberries	1 cup
Strawberries, whole	1-1/4 cups
Tangerine, 8 oz.	2 small
Watermelon, 13-1/2 oz.	
Diced	1-1/4 cups
Slice	1

FRUIT JUICE

BE SURE:

To monitor your blood glucose levels when you drink juice. Fruit juice may cause your blood glucose to rise faster than eating fresh fruit, especially when consumed on an empty stomach. Limit your intake of juice to no more than one meal each day or to times when you are engaging in vigorous activity or treating a low blood glucose.

ITEM	SERVING SIZE
Apple juice, unsweetened	4 oz.
Black cherry juice	3 oz.
Blueberry juice	4 oz.
Cranapple, cocktail	3 oz.
Cranberry juice cocktail	3 oz.
Cranberry, light style	12 oz.
Fruit juice blends	4 oz.
Grape juice, unsweetened	3 oz.
Grapefruit juice, unsweetened	5 oz.
Lemon juice, unsweetened	8 oz.
Orange juice, unsweetened	4 oz.
Peach nectar	3 oz.
Pineapple juice, unsweetened	4 oz.
Pomegranate juice	4 oz.
Prune juice, unsweetened	3 oz.

VEGETABLE CHOICES

BE SURE:
To eat at least 2-1/2 cups of vegetables each day.

WE ENCOURAGE:
Steaming with small amount of water. Portion listed is for cooked serving unless noted otherwise.

ITEM	SERVING SIZE
Artichoke	1/2 medium
Asparagus, cooked	1/2 cup
Bamboo shoots, cooked	1 cup
Bean sprouts	1 cup
Beets, cooked	1/2 cup
Beet greens, cooked	1/2 cup
Broccoli, cooked	1/2 cup
Brussel sprouts, cooked	1/2 cup
Cabbage, cooked	1 cup
Carrots, cooked	1/2 cup
Cauliflower, cooked	1 cup
Celery, raw	1 cup
Collard greens, cooked	1/2 cup
Eggplant	1/2 cup
Green beans, cooked	1/2 cup
Green pepper, raw	1 cup
Jicama, raw	1/2 cup
Kale, cooked	1/2 cup
Kohlrabi, cooked	1/2 cup
Leeks, cooked	1/2 cup
Mushrooms, cooked	1/2 cup
Mustard greens, cooked	1 cup
Okra, cooked	1/2 cup
Onion, raw	1/2 cup
Pea pods (snow peas), ckd	1/2 cup
Radishes	1 cup
Red pepper	1/2 cup
Rutabagas	1/2 cup

BEST CHOICES:
Fresh or frozen vegetables: dark green, leafy or orange. One serving equals 1/2 cup cooked vegetable or 1 cup raw.

One choice provides:
Calories: 25
Carb: 5 gms
Protein: 2 gms
Fat: 0 gms

continued...

VEGETABLE CHOICES *(continued)*

ITEM	SERVING SIZE
*Sauerkraut	1/2 cup
Spinach, cooked	1/2 cup
Squash, cooked	
summer	1/2 cup
spaghetti	1/2 cup
zucchini	1/2 cup
Swiss chard	1 cup
Tomato, 3 oz.	1 small
Tomato, cherry	5 medium
*Tomato, canned	1/2 cup
*Tomato paste	2 Tbsp.
*Tomato sauce, canned	1/3 cup
Turnip greens	1 cup
Turnips, cooked	1/2 cup
Vegetables, mixed	1/2 cup
V-8 juice	1/2 cup
V-8 Splash, diet	1 cup
Wax beans, cooked	1/2 cup
Water chestnuts	1/4 cup

continued...

VEGETABLE CHOICES (continued)

Because of their low carbohydrate and calorie content, the following RAW vegetables may be used liberally.

Alfalfa sprouts	Lettuce, all types
Celery	Mushrooms
Chicory	Parsley
Chinese cabbage	*Pickles (unsweetened)
Cucumber	Pimiento
Endive	Spinach
Escarole	Watercress

*These vegetables are high in sodium (salt). Use low-sodium vegetables, juices and sauces if you are following a low-sodium diet. Fresh and frozen vegetables are lower in sodium than canned vegetables unless the canned product states "no salt added."

MILK CHOICES
NON-FAT SELECTIONS

BE SURE:

You take a calcium supplement if you use less than 2 cups per day for adults, 3-4 cups per day for children.

ITEM	SERVING SIZE
Fat-free milk (skim)	1 cup
Fat-free buttermilk	1 cup
Fat-free Lactaid milk (skim)	1 cup
1/2% milk	1 cup
Fat-free plain yogurt	2/3 cup
Fat-free yogurt, flavored, sweetened with nonnutritive sweetener and fructose	2/3 cup
Powdered, non-fat milk, dry	1/3 cup
Evaporated skim milk	1/2 cup
Fat-free rice milk, plain	1 cup
Fat-free soy milk, plain	1 cup
*Sugar-free hot cocoa mix plus 6 oz. of water	1 cup

> **BEST CHOICES:**
> Non-fat or low-fat
>
> **One choice provides:**
> Calories: 90
> Carb: 12 gms
> Protein: 8 gms
> Fat: 0 gms

Most cocoa mixes do not provide the same amount of calcium as one cup of milk. Mixes which do provide the same amount should indicate on the label that the product contains 30% Daily Value for calcium.

MILK CHOICES
LOW-FAT SELECTIONS

ITEM	SERVING SIZE
1% milk	1 cup
1% buttermilk	1 cup
Low-fat yogurt, plain	1 cup
Low-fat Lactaid milk (1%)	1 cup
Low-fat acidophilus milk	1 cup
Low-fat chocolate milk	1/2 cup
Low-fat rice milk, plain	1 cup
Low-fat soy milk, plain	1 cup
Low-fat soy milk, flavored	3/4 cup

BEST CHOICES: Non-fat or low-fat

One choice provides:
Calories: 105
Carb: 12 gms
Protein: 8 gms
Fat: 3 gms

MILK CHOICES
MEDIUM-AND
HIGH-FAT SELECTIONS

The following milk items should be used sparingly due to their high saturated fat and cholesterol content.

ITEM	SERVING SIZE
2% milk	1 cup
Whole milk	1 cup
Evaporated whole milk	1/2 cup
Goat's milk	1 cup
Kefir	1 cup
Yogurt, plain (made from whole milk)	3/4 cup

One choice provides:
Calories: 120-150
Carb: 12 gms
Protein: 8 gms
Fat: 5-8 gms

Other Carbohydrates

Breakfast Items ITEM	SERVING SIZE	FOOD GROUP	GRAMS CARB	CAL
Nutrigrain Bar	1	2 carbs + 1 fat	27	140
Muffin, bran or corn	1 medium (2 oz.)	1-1/2 carbs + 1 fat	24	160
Weight Watchers Blueberry Muffin	1	2 carbs + 1 fat	37	37
Croissant	1 (2-1/2 oz)	2 carbs + 4 fats	35	300
Doughnut, plain	1 small (1-3/4 oz.)	1-1/2 carbs + 2 fats	25	210
Doughnut, glazed	1 (2 oz.)	2 carbs + 3 fats	29	250
Sweet roll/Danish	1 (2 oz.)	1-1/2 carbs + 2 fats	25	220
Biscuit	1 (1 oz.)	1 carb + 1 fat	13	125
Cornbread, from mix	1 (3 oz.)	2 carbs + 1 fat	36	180
Pancake	2 (4" diam.)	1-1/2 carbs + 1 fat	22	160
Waffle, homemade	1 (7" diam)	2 carbs + 2 fats	26	245
frozen	1 (4" diam.)	1 carb + 1 fat	15	85
Granola, regular	1/4 cup	1 carb + 1 fat	20	125
low-fat	1/4 cup	1 carb	16	80

Desserts

ITEM	SERVING SIZE	FOOD GROUP	GRAMS CARB	CAL
Angel food cake	1/12 of cake	2 carbs	30	160
Brownie, unfrosted	2-inch square	2 carbs + 1 fat	25	205
Cake, unfrosted	2 oz.	2 carbs + 1 fat	35	205
Cake, frosted	2 oz.	3 carbs + 1 fat	40	285
Cupcake, frosted	1 small	2 carbs + 1 fat	28	205
Ice cream				
regular	1/2 cup	1 carb + 2 fat	17	170
light	1/2 cup	1 carb + 2 fat	18	140
no sugar added	1/2 cup	1 carb + 1 fat	15	120
Frozen dessert bars:				
Creamsicle, regular	1 bar	1 carb + 1 fat	20	110
Fruit juice bar	1 bar	1 carb	11	45
No sugar added	1 bar	1/2 carb	6	25
Fudgesicle	1 bar	1 carb	12	60
No sugar added	2 bars	1 carb	19	90
Popsicle	1 bar	1 carb	11	45
Sugar-free	2 bars	1/2 carb	6	30
Ice cream sandwich	1	2 carbs + 1 fat	26	170

continued...

Desserts (continued)

ITEM	SERVING SIZE	FOOD GROUP	GRAMS CARB	CAL
Frozen yogurt				
low-fat	1/2 cup	2 carbs + 1 fat	26	140
fat-free	1/2 cup	2 carbs	29	110
Sherbet, sorbet	1/2 cup	2 carbs	28	120
Pudding:				
sugar-free	1/2 cup	1 carb	11	80
regular	1/2 cup	2 carbs	30	170

Miscellaneous

ITEM	SERVING SIZE	FOOD GROUP	GRAMS CARB	CAL
Jam/Jelly/Honey				
regular	1Tbsp.	1 carb	16	55
Spaghetti sauce	1/2 cup	1 carb + 1 fat	6	135
Sugar	1 Tbsp.	1 carb	12	48
Syrup:				
light	2 Tbsp.	1 carb	12	50
regular	2 Tbsp.	2 carbs	28	110
Yogurt, fruited, regular	1 cup	3 carbs	45	240
French fries	12	1 carb + 1 fat	15	123

Protein List

VERY LEAN SELECTIONS

ITEM	SERVING SIZE
Beef:	
Healthy Choice 97% lean ground beef	1 oz.
*Cheese products, fat-free	1 oz.
shredded	3 Tbsp.
*Cottage cheese, fat-free or 1%	1/4 cup
*Ricotta, fat-free	1 oz.
Dried beans, cooked	1/2 cup = 1 protein + 1 carb
Egg substitute, plain	1/4 cup
Egg whites	2
Fish and seafood: fresh or frozen cod, flounder, haddock, halibut, trout, shrimp, tuna (packed in water), crab, lobster, scallops, imitation crabmeat, clams,	1 oz.
Game: duck or pheasant (no skin), goat, venison, buffalo, ostrich	1 oz.
Hot dog (1 gram fat or less)	1 oz.
Kidney	1 oz.
Poultry: chicken, turkey, or Cornish hen (white meat, no skin)	1 oz.

BEST CHOICES:
Very low fat or low fat selections

One choice provides:
Calories: 35-45
Carb: 0 gms
Protein: 7 gms
Fat: 0-1 gms

* High in sodium

LEAN SELECTIONS

ITEM	SERVING SIZE
Beef:	
USDA Select or Choice grades of flank, round, sirloin, T-bone, tenderloin cuts, ground round	1 oz.
Cheeses	
Cottage cheese, 4.5% fat	1/4 cup
Mozzarella, lite	1 oz.
Parmesan	2 Tbsp.
Fish:	
Herring (uncreamed or *smoked), salmon, tuna canned in oil, drained	1 oz.
oysters	6 medium
sardines	2 medium
*Hot dog (3 grams fat or less)	1 oz.
Lamb:	
roast, chop or leg	1 oz.
Liver	1 oz.
*Luncheon meats: ham, turkey ham, turkey bologna, turkey pastrami, turkey kielbasa	1 oz.
Pork: lean only center loin, fresh ham, loin chop, tenderloin,	
*Canadian bacon	1 oz.
Poultry: chicken, turkey (dark meat, no skin), chicken (white meat, skin), duck or goose (no skin)	1 oz.
Veal:	
lean chop, roast	1 oz.

> **One choice provides:**
> Calories: 55
> Carb: 0 gms
> Protein: 7 gms
> Fat: 3 gms

*High in sodium

MEDIUM-FAT SELECTIONS

ITEM	SERVING SIZE
Beef:	
chuck, flank steak;	
hamburger (90% fat-free), rib	
eye, rump, sirloin, tenderloin	
top and bottom round	1 oz.
*Cheese:	
part-skim mozzarella	1 oz.
part-skim ricotta	1/4 cup
Egg	1
Lamb:	
rib roast, ground	1 oz.
Pork:	
top loin, chop,	
Boston butt, cutlet	1 oz.
Poultry:	
chicken (dark meat,	
with skin) ground chicken	
or turkey	1 oz.
Tempeh	1/4 cup
Tofu	4 oz.
*Turkey sausage, 90% fat-free	1 oz.
Veal: lean, trimmed only,	
loin chop, round	1 oz.

> **One choice provides:**
> Calories: 75
> Carb: 0 gms
> Protein: 7 gms
> Fat: 5 gms

High in sodium

HIGH-FAT SELECTIONS

BE SURE:

To use the protein choices below sparingly, as they are high in saturated fat.

ITEM	SERVING SIZE
Bacon	3 slices
Beef:	
brisket, club and rib steak,	
*corned beef, regular hamburger	
with 20% fat, rib roast,	
short ribs	1 oz.
*Cheese:	
American, blue, brie,	
cheddar, feta,	
Monterey Jack, Swiss	1 oz.
Fish, fried	1 oz.
*Hot dog (beef, pork,	
combination)	1 (10/lb)
Lamb: breast	1 oz.
*Luncheon meat:	
bologna, salami,	
pimento loaf	1 oz.
Peanut butter	1 Tbsp. =
	1 protein
	+ 1 fat
*Pepperoni	1 oz.
Pork:	
spareribs, ground pork,	
pork sausage	1 oz.
Poultry:	
duck (with skin), goose	
(with skin)	1 oz.
Sausage:	
bratwurst, Italian,	
knockwurst, Polish, smoked	1 oz.

> **One choice provides:**
> Calories: 100
> Carb: 0 gms
> Protein: 7 gms
> Fat: 8 gms

High in sodium

Fat List

MONO UN-SATURATED FATS

BE SURE:
When using lower calorie versions of fat choices, use amounts equal to 45 calories for one serving.

ITEM	SERVING SIZE
Avocado, medium	1/8 (1 oz.)
Nondairy creamer, liquid	2 Tbsp.
reduced fat	5 Tbsp.
Nuts:	
almonds, cashews	6
Brazil	2
filberts (hazelnuts)	5
macadamia	3
mixed	6
peanuts, Spanish	20
peanuts, Virginia	10
pecans	4 halves
pignolia (pine nuts)	1 Tbsp.
pistachio	16
Oils: canola, olive, peanut	1 tsp.
*Olives:	
black	8 large
green	10 large
Peanut butter	1/2 Tbsp.
Sesame seeds	1 Tbsp.
Tahini (sesame paste)	2 tsp.

High in sodium

BEST CHOICES:
Monounsaturated fats. However, limit total amount of all types of fat for weight control.

One choice provides:
Calories: 45
Carb: 0 gms
Protein: 0 gms
Fat: 5 gms

POLYUNSATURATED FATS

ITEM	SERVING SIZE
Margarine:	
stick, tub or squeeze	1 tsp.
reduced fat	1 Tbsp.
Mayonnaise	1 tsp.
reduced fat	1 Tbsp.
Mayonnaise-style dressing	2 tsp.
reduced fat	1 Tbsp.
Nuts: walnuts	4 halves
Oils: corn, cottonseed,	
safflower, soy, sunflower	1 tsp.
Salad Dressings, regular:	
*Balsamic vinaigrette	1 Tbsp.
*French, 1000 Island	1 Tbsp.
*Italian	1 Tbsp.
Salad Dressings, reduced calorie:	
*Balsamic vinaigrette	2 Tbsp.
*Italian	2 Tbsp.
*Ranch	1 Tbsp.
^Seeds: pumpkin, sunflower	1 Tbsp.

*High in sodium

SATURATED FATS

BE SURE:

To limit the fat choices below, as they can raise your blood cholesterol levels and increase your risk for heart disease.

ITEM	SERVING SIZE
*Bacon, cooked	1 slice
Bacon grease	1 tsp.
Butter: stick	1 tsp.
whipped	2 tsp.
reduced fat	1 Tbsp.
Chitterlings	2 Tbsp. (1/2 oz.)
Coconut, shredded	2 Tbsp.
Coconut milk	1 Tbsp.
Cream:	
half & half	2 Tbsp.
heavy	1 Tbsp.
light	1-1/2 Tbsp.
whipped	1 Tbsp.
whipped, pressurized	1/4 cup
Cream cheese, regular	1 Tbsp.
reduced fat	2 Tbsp.
Oils: coconut or palm	1 tsp.
Salt pork	1/4 oz.
Shortening or lard	1 tsp.
Sour cream: regular	2 Tbsp.
reduced fat	3 Tbsp.

*High in sodium

"Free" Foods List

> **BE SURE:**
> A "free" food is any food or drink that contains less than 20 calories per serving, and no more than 5 grams of carbohydrate per serving. Limit those free foods that have a serving size (on page 124) to 3 per day, and spread out your use of free foods over the day. Items marked with an asterisk (*) are high in sodium.
>
> ## GENERAL:
>
> *Bouillon, broth, or consommé
> Chewing gum, sugar-free
> Cocoa powder
> Non-caloric diet soft drinks, unsweetened
> seltzer waters
> Coffee (black)
> Tea
> Cranberries (unsweetened)
> Extracts
> Gelatin mixes, sugar-free
> Herbs, seasonings, spices
> Lemon/lime juice
> Lemon/lime/orange rind
> *Pickles (unsweetened)
> Postum (limit to 3 cups daily)
> *Soy sauce, steak sauce
> Sugar substitutes (acesulfame-K, aspartame, saccharin, sucralose)
> *Tabasco sauce
> Vinegar

Many fat-free choices contain one or more types of sugar. The amount of sweetener is small; however, the portion used should be no more than the amount listed on this page or no more than 20 calories per serving approximately three times per day. Always read the labels carefully. Remember that fat-free does not mean carbohydrate-free.

ITEM	SERVING SIZE
Bran	1 Tbsp.
*Catsup	1 Tbsp.
Cream Cheese:	
fat-free	1 Tbsp.
*Gravy:	
fat-free	2 Tbsp.
Hard candy or mints,	
sugar-free	3 or less
Jams:	
light jam or jelly	2 tsp.
Mayonnaise:	
fat-free	1 Tbsp.
reduced-fat	1 tsp.
Margarine:	
fat-free spread	4 Tbsp.
reduced-fat spread	1 tsp.
Butter substitutes	
Butter Buds	1 Tbsp.
Molly McButter	2 tsp.
Non-stick sprays	3-second spray
*Mustard	1 Tbsp.
Popsicles, no sugar added	1 bar
Salad dressing:	
fat-free or low fat	1 Tbsp.
Salsa	1/4 cup
Sour cream:	
fat-free or reduced fat	1 Tbsp.
Syrup, sugar-free	2 Tbsp.
Taco sauce	1 Tbsp.
Whipped topping:	
regular	1 Tbsp.
light or fat-free	2 Tbsp.
Yogurt, plain	2 Tbsp.

*High in sodium

> **One choice =**
> a free food
>
> **Remember:**
> If you have more than 3 servings of free foods, you'll need to count the carbs.

Combination Foods List

Many foods are made up of several food groups. These mixed foods can be incorporated into your meal plan by substituting them for choices from more than one food group.

*CANNED SOUP

ITEM	SERVING SIZE	FOOD GROUP	GRAMS CARB	CAL
Rice or noodle with broth prepared with water	1 cup	1 carb	15	100
Cream soup Made with water	1 cup	1 carb, 1 fat	15	110
Clam Chowder, New England style	1 cup	1 carb, 2 fats	20	200
Lentil with ham, ready to serve	1 cup	2 carbs, 1 protein,	30	145
Minestrone	1 cup	1 carb	20	100
Split pea with ham	1 cup	2 carb, 1 protein	28	165
Tomato, made with water	1 cup	1 carb	19	100
Vegetable, made with water	1 cup	1 carb	15	80

*High in sodium

ITEM	SERVING SIZE	FOOD GROUP	GRAMS CARB	CAL
Beef stew, homemade	1 cup	1 carb 1 protein	19	112
Chicken potpie, frozen	1 cup	3 carbs, 2 proteins, 6 fats	44	500
Chili with meat and beans, homemade	1 cup	1 1/2 carbs, 3 proteins, 2 fats	22	255
Lasagna, homemade	2-1/2 x 2-1/2 x 1-3/4 in.	2 carbs, 3 proteins, 1 vegetable, 2 fat	35	215
Macaroni & cheese, made from package	1 cup	3 carbs, 2 proteins, 1 fat	45	390
Pizza, Cheese	1/4 of 12 in. diameter	2 carbs, 2 proteins, 3 fats	29	320
Ravioli, canned	1 cup (7 oz.)	2 carbs, 1 protein, 2 fats	35	240
Spaghetti with meat balls, canned	1 cup	2 carbs, 1 protein, 2 fats	32	250

*High in sodium unless specially prepared without salt.

Fast Foods List

Guidelines for Fast Foods

The list below gives you information on typical fast foods. For more specific information, ask for nutrition information when you are in a fast food restaurant, or check the restaurant's web site. Use these guidelines for making healthier choices from fast food menus.

▲ Look out for hidden fats. Deep fat frying and batter coating can double or triple the number of calories.

▲ Many food items contain ingredients from more than one food group. Fat is often a second ingredient. Portion sizes may need to be reduced in order to fit some of these food items into your meal plan.

▲ Menu items such as pie, milkshakes, regular sodas, and even juices contain large amounts of carbohydrate and can significantly increase your blood glucose. Talk with your dietitian regarding how to include such choices.

▲ Due to high fat and sodium content, fast foods should be eaten only occasionally.

ITEM	SERVING SIZE	FOOD GROUP	GRAMS CARB	CAL
Burrito, beef	1 regular	3 carbs, 2 proteins, 3 fats	50	390
Cheeseburger	1 regular	2 carbs, 2 proteins, 2 fats	35	310
Chicken, fried, drumstick and wing	1 each	1 carb, 3 proteins, 4 fats	9	290

ITEM	SERVING SIZE	FOOD GROUP	GRAMS CARB	CAL
Chicken pieces	6	1 carb, 2 proteins, 3 fats	15	250
Chicken sandwich	1	3 carbs, 2 proteins, 4 fats	41	420
Egg sandwich	1	2 carbs, 2 proteins, 2 fats	30	290
French fries, med.	1 serving	3 carbs, 3 fats	47	350
Fried fish sandwich	1	3 carbs, 2 proteins, 4 fats	42	400
Hamburger, regular	1	2 carbs, 2 proteins, 2 fats	33	260
Hamburger, large	1	3 carbs, 3 proteins, 4 fats	40	420
Pizza, cheese, thin crust (12")	1 slice	1 carb, 1 protein, 2 fats	21	200
Taco, beef	1 regular	1 carb, 1 protein, 2 fats	13	170

Food Lists for Vegetarian Meal Plans

CARBOHYDRATE FOODS

ITEM	SERVING SIZE
Starch: Grains / Breads / Starchy Vegetables	
Serving = 1 carb (15 g carb, 3 g protein)	
Pita bread	1/2 of 2 oz. loaf
Corn/flour tortilla, 6"	1
Miso	3 Tbsp.
Cooked grains	
Bulgur	1/2 cup
Oat bran	1/4 cup
Buckwheat	1/2 cup
Couscous	1/3 cup
Barley	1/3 cup
Quinoa	1/3 cup
Wheat berries	2/3 cup
Brown rice	1/3 cup
Wild rice	1/2 cup
Milk:	
Serving = 1 carb and – 2 fats (15 g carb, 8 g protein, 2-10 g fat)	
Goat milk	1 cup
Kefir	1 cup
Soy milk	1 cup
Rice milk	1 cup
Acidophilus milk	1 cup
Buttermilk	1 cup
Vegetables:	
"free" for 1-2 servings – 5 g carb (15 g carb for 3 servings)	
Bamboo shoots	1/2 cup
Greens	1/2 cup
Seaweed	1 oz.
Celeriac, raw	1/2 cup
Jicama, raw	1/2 cup
Sprouts	1/2 cup
Endive	1 medium head

MEAT SUBSTITUTES / PROTEIN FOODS

ITEM	SERVING SIZE
Serving = 1 protein (0 g carb, 7 g protein, 0-5 g fat)	
Tofu, firm	1/2 cup (4 oz.)
Vegetarian breakfast links	1 link (1 oz)*
Egg substitute	1/4 cup
Vegetarian breakfast patties	1 patty (1.3 oz)*
Soy cheese	1 oz.
Vegetarian hotdog	1 hotdog (1.5 oz)*

Some vegetarian meat substitutes may also contain carbohydrate

Beans (cooked):
Serving = 1 carb + 1 lean protein (15 g carb, 7 g protein)

Black-eyed peas	1/2 cup
Lentils	1/2 cup
Black beans	1/2 cup
Navy, kidney, pinto beans	1/3 cup
Refried beans	1/2 cup
Chick peas, garbanzo beans	1/3 cup
Lima beans	1/2 cup
Split peas	1/3 cup

Nuts/Seeds:
Serving = 1 protein + 2-3 fats (0 g carb, 7 g protein, 10-15 g fat)

Almonds, pecans, peanuts	1/4 cup
Walnuts	16 – 20 halves
Pine nuts, pignolias	2 Tbsp
Pistachios	1/4 cup (1 oz.)
Pumpkin or squash seeds	1/4 cup
Sesame or sunflower seeds	1/4 cup

FAT FOODS

ITEM	SERVING SIZE
Serving = 1 fat (0 g carb, 5 g fat)	
Almond butter	1 Tbsp = 2 fat
Flax seed oil	1 tsp = 1 fat
Cashew butter	1 Tbsp = 2 fat
Peanut oil	1 tsp = 1 fat
Sesame butter, tahini	1 Tbsp = 2 fat

COMBINATION FOODS

Bean and cheese tostada	1 tostada (5 oz) 2 carbs, 1 protein, 3 fat
Falafel	3 patties (3 oz) 1 carb, 1 protein, 4 fat 2" diam.
Hummus	1/2 cup 1 carb, 1 protein, 2 fat
Tempeh	1/2 cup 1 carb, 2 protein
Textured vegetable protein	3/4 oz. 1/2 carb, 1 protein
Tofu-based ice cream	1/2 cup 1 carb, 2 fat
Vegetarian chili	2/3 cup 1 carb, 3 protein
Vegetarian "garden" burger	1 patty (2.5 oz) 1 carb, 1 protein
Vegetarian soy burger	1 patty (2.5 oz) 1/2 carb, 2 protein
Wheat germ, toasted	1/2 cup 1 carb, 1 protein, 2 fat

*Depending on the brand or preparation method, these foods may have additional fat

NOTES